THE CARDIAC PATIENT

THE CARDIAC PATIENT

George W. Paterson

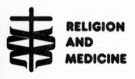

RELIGION AND MEDICINE

Glen W. Davidson, Editor

AUGSBURG PUBLISHING HOUSE
MINNEAPOLIS, MINNESOTA

THE CARDIAC PATIENT

Contents

Foreword

My heart is my most carefully monitored organ. At times I forget about it, taking its vital functions for granted. But when I overexert myself physically, or become frustrated or angry, or even when I feel lonely, I become all too aware of how much I depend on this muscle and I realize that its function is central to my personal identity.

Modern man is not alone in referring to the heart and its functions as symbolic of one's life. Some tribal peoples of the world interpreted the heart as the oracle of communication with their gods. In biblical times, the heart was understood as the central and unifying organ of personal life, of wisdom and morality. Today, we speak of the heart as the seat of personality. For example, when we say one is cold-hearted, we mean that he is calculating, intolerant and lacking in compassion. When we say he is warm-hearted, we mean the person is forgiving, tolerant, and generous. We use such terms as broken-hearted, sick-at-heart, and heartless. We are well aware that some people who have "heart trouble" go through a personality change and become emotionally brittle, cranky, and intolerant.

This book tells about the heart, how it functions, and what happens when it malfunctions because of disease. More important, the author helps us understand the task of reinterpreting our personal identities in the face of cardiac malfunction.

This book is included in the RELIGION AND MEDICINE SERIES to help people facing heart disease with their efforts to remain whole despite cardiac malfunction. It is a book for those who seek spiritual insight, written by an author who has faced heart disease in his own family.

Dr. Paterson is an Associate Professor in the School of Religion and College of Medicine, and Associate Director of Pastoral Services of the University of Iowa Hospitals and Clinics. He received his Bachelor of Divinity degree from Drew University in 1955 and his Doctor of Philosophy degree from the University of Iowa in 1969. In 1975, he wrote another book for the Series: *Helping Your Handicapped Child* which has appeared in both English and Swedish.

Glen W. Davidson, Ph.D.
Professor and Chairman
Department of Medical Humanities
Southern Illinois University
School of Medicine

A Word to the Reader

Writing this book has turned out to be an unusually difficult task. When I was invited to do a book on the spiritual dimensions of heart disease, I accepted with eagerness, for this was a subject which had long held keen interest for me. As a pastor and later a hospital chaplain I had ministered to many persons suffering from heart disease during the past twenty years; moreover, my family has had considerable experience with this problem. Both my father and his only brother died of heart disease while in their fifties. Writing this book would be an opportunity to explore in depth a topic that concerned me personally as well as professionally.

However, as I began to review the literature on the heart and its disorders, something unexpected happened. I began finding all kinds of reasons for putting off work on the book. Of course the pressure of a busy schedule of teaching and pastoral work in the hospital provided a ready excuse for delaying research on heart disease. But there was more to the delay than simple lack of time. I found myself becoming unusually aware of minor aches, pains, and troubling sensations in my chest. My physician examined me thoroughly and re-assured me that I was in good health, but the awareness persisted. I wondered, "Are these feelings normal? Am I making them up? Did I always have them, but just didn't notice them?" About this time a close relative, five years younger than I, suffered a very unexpected heart attack. Now I was forced to recognize why I had been putting off work on this book: I was anxious and apprehensive about my own heart. The more I read about the heart and its disorders, the more my personal anxiety over heart disease came to the surface.

I mention this because I believe my own reaction to the subject is a very common one. Heart disease is a subject about which many of us feel a great deal of anxiety, and rightly so. For that reason, those who read this book may find, as I have in writing it, that it is hard to stick with the subject, and easy to put aside. By all means take a break from reading it if you find it disturbing. But don't let yourself ignore the subject of heart disease for that reason. It is too real and too widespread to be ignored. Further, if we will seek to understand it, there is a great deal we can do to prevent it, treat it, and if necessary, live with it.

Few families in the United States have not felt the impact of heart disease. In 1974, 1,036,560 persons died as a result of cardiovascular disease in the United States; this figure represents 53 % of the deaths from all causes in the nation for that year. During that same period, 3,490,000 persons suffered heart attacks. The total yearly cost to our society from heart disease has been estimated at $20 billion; this includes the cost of physician and nursing services, research, the construction of special care units, and wages lost by persons affected. Whether or not we ourselves expect to suffer from one of this group of diseases, none of us can afford to ignore their impact on our lives. Yet we would often prefer not to think about them.

This book is not, however, about heart disease as such, but about the spiritual problems—and opportunities—which confront heart patients and their families. The word *spiritual* is so often misused and misunderstood that it requires an explanation. To some persons it means the opposite of all that is material or physical. Something that is spiritual is thought to be intangible, immaterial, or ethereal. To others the term signifies a certain refinement of taste, the opposite of all that is earthy or crude. A spiritual person is one who prefers poetry to football, or string quartets to jazz. Still other persons use the term to indicate concerns that are predominantly inner- or other-worldly. In this sense, a spiritual person may be one who spends more time in prayer and meditation than in political activity. I do not intend to use the term in any of these ways; rather, I intend to use it to refer to the *wholeness* and *unity* of our personal existence, and to the integration of the many dimensions that make up that wholeness. To me the word *spiritual* includes the biological dimensions of life as well as the religious, the physical as well as the intellectual. It encompasses our feelings, relationships, attitudes and values, our goals and aspirations, our ethical principles and behavior, our religious beliefs and practices—all that makes us truly, distinctively and fully human. The central concern of this book is to ask, how can persons meet the threat of heart disease and yet retain their grasp of that which makes them truly human beings?

A number of persons have generously taken the time to read and respond to this manuscript. I am grateful for the critical and constructive suggestions of Roland Seboldt, John Saeger, Glen Davidson, and Ernest O. Theilen, M.D. Colleen Lewis has typed and re-typed the various drafts with unfailing patience and accuracy. In the end, however, I must take responsibility for both form and the content of the book.

Finally, a word about the case material. In two instances (Ken Madison and Vivian Hellstrom) the patients are composites rather than actual persons. The material is, I trust, typical enough to illustrate the general features of each situation. In other cases, the patients are real, but fictitious names have been used to protect their privacy.

1

The Wounded Heart

In order for us to explore the spiritual dimensions of heart disease, it is necessary to begin with a very brief and non-technical review of how the heart functions in health and illness. Although this chapter may not make the most enjoyable reading, I hope you will bear with me, for unless we have some understanding of the way our bodies function, we cannot deal realistically with the threat of illness. And if a spiritual perspective really does emphasize the wholeness and unity of our being, it must include an appreciation of that mysterious and amazing physical organism which is an essential part of our being.

The heart functions as a pump which keeps the tissues of our body supplied with the oxygen which is essential to their survival. It consists of a hollow mass of muscle containing four chambers. Two of these, called *atria*, serve as holding chambers to receive the blood which enters the heart through the veins. The other two chambers, called *ventricles*, contract to propel blood from the heart to other parts of the body. Actually, the heart consists of two pumps, one on the right and the other on the left side. The right atrium receives blood returning from all parts of the body except the lungs, and releases it to the right ventricle, which then ejects this blood through the pulmonary artery to the lungs. There carbon dioxide is released and the blood is recharged with life-sustaining oxygen. The oxygenated blood then flows back through the pulmonary vein into the left atrium of the heart, from which it flows into the left ventricle, which in turn propels it through the aorta to all organs and tissues of the body. All of this takes place on the average of 70 times per minute in the normal adult, and results in the circulation of approximately a gallon and a half of blood throughout the entire body in a minute. Our lives depend utterly on this process, which began eight months before we were born and continues every moment of every day as long as we live. If it is interrupted for even a few minutes the brain, which is vulnerable to oxygen deprivation, will cease to function and death will follow soon.

However, a number of disorders can interfere with the normal healthy functioning of the heart and cause it to fail. Heart failure occurs when for any of several reasons the heart is unable to pump sufficient blood to meet the demands of the other tissues of the body. When the left ventricle fails, rising pressures in this chamber may be reflected backward into the lungs, causing congestion and shortness of breath. If the right ventricle fails, congestion will occur throughout the body, and will cause a watery swelling in the tissues called edema or dropsy. Heart failure may result from a variety of causes including poor blood supply through the coronary arteries, abnormal or diseased valves within the heart, high blood pressure, and other less common disorders. The person suffering from heart failure may be treated by limiting the amount of physical exertion he can undertake to reduce the load on the heart, giving digitalis to strengthen the contractions, restricting the salt in his diet, and prescribing diuretic medications to remove fluid from the body tissues.

Coronary Heart Disease

One of the most common of the disorders to affect the heart is *coronary heart disease*. This is the disease which can cause "heart attacks," from which nearly 3½ million Americans suffered in 1974. Approximately 17% of these attacks —683,100—were fatal. The next most frequent cause of death, cancer, was responsible for only about half as many fatalities (346,930).

The most common condition associated with coronary heart disease is *atherosclerosis* of the coronary arteries. It is these vessels which encircle the heart like a crown ("corona") and provide the blood supply for the heart muscle itself. The term *atherosclerosis* refers to the narrowing or blocking of these arteries by fatty deposits within the arterial walls. In time, scar tissue forms within these deposits; later the deposits may become calcified, and a hard, chalk-like plaque forms which can block the flow of blood through the vessels. Also, wherever a vessel is constricted, there is a greater likelihood that the circulation may be interrupted by the presence of a blood clot, causing *coronary thrombosis*. Since the heart muscle uses about 80% of the oxygen provided by its blood supply, there is little reserve oxygen available in case blood supply is reduced. Whenever increased activity causes the heart to work harder, the muscle demands more oxygen, and the coronary arteries supply an increased volume of blood. The tissues of the heart are therefore quite vulnerable to any reduction or stoppage in the supply of blood. In other parts of the body there are numerous cross connections or collaterals between arteries, so that if one vessel is blocked, the tissues it serves can be supplied by others. The arteries which supply the heart muscle, however, possess relatively few collaterals. Thus the blocking of a coronary artery by plaque or by a blood clot may very quickly deprive a given area of the heart muscle of its essential oxygen, and bring about the death of that portion of tissue.

Coronary heart disease gives rise to two main types of illness. When the coronary arteries are narrowed but not completely blocked, the heart may function normally at rest or with moderate activity. But when increased exertion makes unusually heavy demands on the muscle, its oxygen supply will fall near or even below the minimum level required for continued functioning. In such cases the person is likely to experience a characteristic disturbance which is variously described as pain, pressure, choking, or constriction in the chest, and which is known as *angina pectoris*. It may be caused by increased physical exertion, eating a large meal, or a high degree of emotional tension, especially intense fear or anger. Angina pectoris is the earliest and mildest form of coronary heart disease, and can usually be relieved in a few moments by rest, the use of nitroglycerin tablets, or both. Certain other drugs may also be prescribed by the physician for the treatment of angina; and for some patients, a surgical procedure known as an aorto-coronary bypass graft may be recommended (see Chapter IV).

The other type of illness to which coronary heart disease can give rise is known by the medical term, *myocardial infarction,* which to most of us means simply, heart attack. When the blood supply to a given area of the heart is completely shut off, that portion of the muscle dies. This is a life-threatening situation which demands immediate and skilled medical intervention. The necessity of prompt treatment for heart attack victims is revealed by studies which show that of those persons who suffer fatal heart attacks, half or more do so before reaching a hospital. However, those who receive appropriate treatment have an excellent chance of surviving their infarct—85% or better.

The usual symptom of myocardial infarction is severe chest pain, which is not relieved by rest or nitroglycerin as is the pain of angina. This pain may occur in a person who has had few or no previous symptoms of heart disease. It may spread to the arms, neck, and jaw, and is sometimes accompanied by perspiration, nausea, vomiting, or shortness of breath. In some instances a myocardial infarction may produce no symptoms at all, and may only be discovered indirectly at a later time.

Persons suspected of having a heart attack should be taken to a hospital immediately, since numerous possibly fatal complications which require skilled medical intervention may develop during the first several days. Even after the patient has survived the initial crisis period he will need to remain in the hospital under close medical supervision for another one to two weeks. When a portion of heart muscle dies from lack of oxygen, it must heal over and form scar tissue. This process requires a period of rest, after which the physician may permit a gradual increase in the patient's activity.

Although the ultimate causes of coronary disease are still unknown, investigators agree that several factors are known to increase the risk of infarction. Among these are hypertension; elevated levels of cholesterol in the blood; cigarette smoking, which reduces the air-exchange capacity of the lungs; and diabetes. A non-smoking man who is free of diabetes, whose blood pressure is normal, and who has normal levels of fat in the bloodstream is thought to have only one chance in twenty of suffering a heart attack before age 65. If any one of these risk factors is present, however, his chances double; and if two of these factors are present, his chances escalate to one in two! A number of other factors are generally thought to increase the likelihood of coronary disease, though their role has yet to be proven. A family history of coronary disease; obesity (10 to 20% over one's ideal weight calculated for ages 20 to 21 years); a high degree of emotional tension or life stress (especially the "type A" personality pattern discussed in Chapter II); and lack of regular daily exercise are all characteristics frequently associated with the occurrence of heart attacks. It is also agreed that sex and age make a significant difference. Coronary artery disease is rarely found in women before the onset of menopause; but women age 65 show as high an incidence as men of the same age. Another well-known study shows that men in their fifties are four times as likely to have a heart attack as those twenty years younger.

Disorders of Heart Rhythm

Another disorder often associated with coronary disease is a disturbance or irregularity in the heartbeat *(arrhythmia)*. The seventy-times-per-minute beat of the normal heart is activated by the heart's own internal pacemaker, called the sinus node, which is located in the right atrium. An electrical impulse which originates here travels through special conduction pathways to stimulate the cells in the walls of the ventricles. The normal heart rate may be altered by vigorous exercise, hormones, drugs, and also by injury or disease. Fortunately the heart is well provided with emergency back-up systems. If the sinus node should fail, another center, the atrio-ventricular node, will take over and drive the heart at a slower rate. If this center fails, certain cells in the ventricles will assume the task of regulating the heartbeat, but at a still slower rate. The person experiencing a heart rhythm disorder may be aware of skipped beats, palpitation or fluttering in the chest, faintness or dizziness; or, the disorder may produce no noticeable sensation. Some arrhythmias occur in otherwise normal, healthy individuals and require no specific medical treatment. Others may appear as a consequence of other types of heart disease and may be so life-threatening that immediate intervention is demanded. Irregularities in heart rhythm are one of the serious complications that may appear during the early stages following a heart attack, and constitute one important reason why the victim of an infarction should be hospitalized at once.

Three common disorders of heart rhythm are extra beats, very slow heartbeat, and very rapid heartbeat. Extra beats may or may not indicate heart disease, but should always be evaluated by a physician, especially when they produce disturbing symptoms such as palpitation, chest pain, or shortness of breath. Slow heart rate may also occur in normal persons as well as those with heart disease. One frequent cause of this disorder is *heart block*, a condition in which there is an interference in the passage of the electrical impulse which regulates the heartbeat somewhere along the conduction pathways. When the block is complete, the heart will continue to beat, driven by cells in the walls of the ventricles, but at a rate of only 20 to 40 beats per minute. In this situation, the physician will normally use an artificial pacemaker either temporarily or permanently to stimulate the heart electronically and restore its normal rhythm.

A long flexible tube or catheter is passed through a vein in the arm or neck into the heart itself. Electrodes at the tip of this tube are then placed in contact with the inner wall of the ventricle so as to transmit an electrical impulse to the muscle. If the pacemaker is to be used permanently a battery will be implanted under the skin of the patient's chest or abdomen to serve as a power source. Although this battery will need to be replaced surgically every few years, in other aspects the patient may be able to carry on a nearly normal life.

Very rapid heartbeat may arise in either the atria or the ventricles. If the rhythm is rapid but regular, the condition is known as *tachycardia;* if the contractions are random, disorganized, and ineffective it is known as *fibrillation*. The most critical of such disorders is *ventricular fibrillation*, in which the heart muscle completely fails in its pumping capacity. Circulation ceases, blood pressure falls to zero, and loss of consciousness and death follow very quickly unless the heart is immediately "defibrillated" by electric countershock. Identical consequences are produced by *cardiac arrest*, in which the heart comes to a complete standstill. Death occurs in minutes unless the heart is restarted by cardiac massage and artificial respiration, or by electric shock.

Besides the methods listed above, the physician may employ a variety of medications in treating arrhythmias, depending on the nature and location of the disorder. In some cases the patient may need to discontinue certain other medications which can themselves produce disturbances of heart rhythm, or to reduce his or her intake of coffee, tobacco, or alcohol.

Hypertensive Heart Disease

Hypertension or high blood pressure is still another condition responsible for heart disease. Blood pressure is measured in two figures, for example, 120/80. The top figure represents the peak pressure in the blood vessels (measured in millimeters of mercury) when the heart is contracting to force blood into the arteries. The lower figure represents the pressure maintained between contractions by the elastic "recoil" of the arteries. The former is called the *systolic,* and the latter the *diastolic* pressure. Blood pressure varies considerably, both from person to person, and within the same person depending on the time of day, rate of physical activity, and the person's emotional state. Nevertheless, physicians can state a normal range for both the systolic and diastolic pressures. For example, in most adults a systolic pressure in the range of 100 to 140 would be considered normal, as would a diastolic pressure of 60 to 90.

Blood pressure can be consistently elevated for numerous reasons. One common cause of systolic hypertension is hardening of the arteries, or arteriosclerosis. This relatively benign form of high blood pressure may occur in older persons whose blood vessels have lost some of their natural capacity to expand when blood is ejected from the heart. A more serious condition exists when both systolic and diastolic pressures are elevated. When this occurs, the left side of the heart must pump constantly against increased resistance; if this situation continues over a long period of time, the heart muscle may wear out and heart failure will follow.

This type of high blood pressure may be the result of certain other abnormal conditions in the body, such as various types of kidney disease and tumors of the adrenal gland. Many cases of high blood pressure, however, are diagnosed as "essential hypertension," which simply means there is no other known cause. In addition to causing heart disease, untreated hypertension can also result in damage to the brain and the kidneys. Fortunately, most cases of high blood pressure can now be treated successfully by one or more of a variety of drugs. Although these drugs do not cure the condition, they control it over long periods of time and thus permit the person to enjoy a reasonably healthy and normal life.

Infectious and Valvular Heart Disease

Like any other organ of the body, the heart is subject to infections and to inflammation. Disease which attacks the sack of tissue which surrounds the heart is referred to as *pericarditis;* if the heart muscle is affected, the disease is known as *myocarditis.* When the inner lining of the heart is involved the condition is called *endocarditis.*

Valvular heart disease may occur as a consequence of rheumatic fever, an acute inflammatory process which sometimes appears in the wake of a particular kind of streptococcal infection which usually attacks the nose and throat. Rheumatic fever can result in permanent damage to the heart by causing scar tissue to form on any of several valves that control the flow of blood within it. These valves may become narrowed or stenotic, so that not enough blood flows through; or they may become leaky (regurgitant), allowing blood to flow back into a chamber from which it has been expelled. In either event, the heart must work harder to supply the body tissues with a sufficient volume of blood. Over a long period of time this condition can lead to a gradual wearing out of the muscle and eventually to heart failure.

Fortunately, not all streptococcal infections result in rheumatic fever, and not all rheumatic fever results in heart disease. About one out of a hundred persons suffering from streptococcal infection will develop rheumatic fever, and about half of these will be affected by heart disease. However, the prompt diagnosis and treatment of such infections by a physician is a wise preventive measure against the possibility of future heart disease.

Congenital Heart Disease

One final type of heart disease remains to be discussed. For reasons that are not well understood, about one in every thousand babies has a congenital or inborn abnormality of the heart. Since many of these children do not survive their first year, the frequency of inborn heart defects in children of one year or older is about one in 3,000. In some children, this disorder will be detected by the presence of a heart murmur; in others, by a characteristic blue color of the skin called *cyanosis*. The color is produced by blood which has been allowed to pass from the veins through the heart and out into the body again without returning to the lungs to be oxygenated. In some children the abnormality may not show itself in either of these ways, and may only be discovered when the child is older.

Some of the more common defects will be mentioned briefly. *Septal defects* consist of holes in the wall separating the right from the left side of the heart. These may occur between either the atria, or the ventricles, and vary both in size and severity. In *patent ductus arteriosus,* an opening between the aorta and pulmonary artery allows the blood to bypass the lungs. This opening is present in all babies before birth but normally closes during the first few weeks of life. *Coarctation of the aorta* involves a constriction of the artery which carries blood from the heart, and causes extra work for the left ventricle. *Stenosis* of the pulmonary or aortic valves is a condition of narrowing that obstructs the flow of blood out of the heart. *Tetralogy of Fallot* is the name given to a complex defect involving both a ventricular septal defect and pulmonary stenosis. *Transposition of the great vessels* occurs when the aorta and the pulmonary artery originate in the wrong ventricles. In this abnormality, blue or venous blood is pumped from the right ventricle back to the body, while pink or oxygenated blood circulates from the left side of the heart to the lungs and back again.

Today many congenital heart defects can be repaired safely and successfully by surgery. In some cases it may be possible to operate while the infant is very small; in others the surgery may be safely postponed until the child is five years or older. With the rapid advances in cardiac surgery of the past ten years, many parents whose child has an inborn heart abnormality have reason to hope that through skilled medical intervention their child may be able to lead a normal, healthy, and active life.

For many of you this chapter has not been easy or pleasant reading. Nor has it been easy to write. The subject of heart disease can be both frightening and depressing. But allow me to remind you of two things. First, for most of us, and for most of our lives, the heart functions with amazing effectiveness and dependability. As the ancient Hebrew poet observed, we are "fearfully and wonderfully made" (Psalm 139:14, KJV). Second, even when disease does strike the heart, there is much that modern medicine can do to strengthen, relieve, renew and heal this life-sustaining organ. In the remainder of this book we will explore some ways in which medical science and intelligent religious faith can work together for the benefit of those people who become "sick at heart."

2

Preventing Coronary Heart Disease

The preceding chapter has sketched a rather somber picture. Yet that picture is far from hopeless, for there is much that can be done to prevent cardiovascular disorders. Our concern in this chapter is to see how persons can protect their health and avert the threat of needless or untimely coronary heart disease.

The importance of preventing heart disease should be clear by now. To the individual, heart disease can mean disability, premature death, substantial loss of income, heavy medical and hospital bills, loss of time from job or profession, inability to carry on family responsibilities, and feelings of anxiety, depression, boredom, and uselessness. Deeply religious people who view life as a calling from God may experience heart disease as a crisis in their vocation of service to God and neighbor. The importance to society of preventing heart disease should likewise be clear. Heart disease causes an enormous loss of human potential that is desperately needed in government, business, education, the arts, social service, and many other crucial areas. Think what we could do to improve the quality of life for all persons in our nation if we could recover a portion of the 19.5 billion dollars, or the 26 million person/days of productive work that are lost each year because of heart disease.

What can we do to prevent heart disease? Some kinds probably cannot be prevented, or may yield only to massive public health measures. For example, the widespread inoculation of children against rubella should eventually reduce the incidence of inborn heart defects. However, it is unlikely that we will ever succeed in eliminating *all* congenital heart disease; and in any event, those persons already unfortunate enough to have been born with it will not be helped directly by such programs. Further, since the most dramatic advances in medical science cannot be expected to make our bodies immortal, it is reasonable to suppose that heart disease will continue to be a common cause of death among older persons who have completed their normal span of life. In spite of these limitations, much heart disease could either be avoided or at least postponed to the natural end-stage of life if persons would observe some sound principles of preventive medicine. In particular, the threat of coronary heart disease could be reduced by proper attention to a number of factors that are known to increase its risk. We shall consider these under two major headings: first, the *physiological* risk factors; and second, the *social* and *emotional* factors that contribute to coronary heart disease.

Physiological Risk Factors

Several physiological factors are known to be associated with the presence of coronary heart disease. One of these is untreated *hypertension* (high blood pressure). Although the reasons for this relationship are not yet fully clear, the fact of it has been demonstrated beyond reasonable doubt. For example, it has been shown that a persistent elevation of the blood pressure above 150/90 speeds the development of disease in the coronary arteries. The problem is complicated by the fact that many persons who have high blood pressure do not experience any disagreeable symptoms. It is often hard to persuade them that they must take medicine daily for a disease that gives no outward signs of its presence. One prominent team of cardiologists has observed that most heart patients are so caught up in the present that they can't be bothered with consequences that will not appear for perhaps another ten years. Indeed, the hypertensive person sometimes feels at his best when his pressures are elevated. Nevertheless, the long-term effects of untreated high blood pressure can be disastrous.

Another condition that adds to the risk of coronary disease is *diabetes,* especially when it is inadequately controlled by diet and medication. As with hypertension, the mechanisms responsible for the association between coronary disease and diabetes are not completely understood, but the positive correlation is unmistakable. Not all diabetics, of course, will develop heart disease, but the presence of the disease definitely increases the risk of damage to the coronary arteries.

A third risk factor on which medical researchers are agreed is a *high level of fats* in the blood, either in the form of cholesterol, triglycerides, or both. Since cholesterol is the most frequently used index of blood fat levels, our discussion will focus on it. Epidemiological studies have shown that in areas where cholesterol levels are as low as 150 mg. per ml. of blood serum, coronary artery disease is rare; but where they range as high as 285 mg. per ml., a large proportion of the population shows signs of coronary atherosclerosis. Other studies have indicated this variation is not determined by race. Some investigators report that the risk of coronary disease is three times as great for men whose cholesterol runs above 260 as for those in whom it is less than 180. Why and how does an elevation of cholesterol in the bloodstream lead to heart disease? Apparently it contributes to the formation of plaque which can eventually block the coronary arteries and cut off blood supply to a portion of the heart muscle. Laboratory studies have shown that when an artery is damaged it heals with a very small scar *unless* excess cholesterol is present in the diet. Then the size of the scar is increased several times over. Some physicians believe the coronary arteries are subject to an unusual amount of stress and minor damage as a result of the constant twisting and turning they receive from the heart muscle. If this is true, it can be seen that they would also be especially vulnerable to the formation of scar tissue in persons whose cholesterol is high.

But what causes cholesterol to be elevated? In some persons this condition is the result of a hereditary disease known as hypercholesterolemia. In many others, however, high levels of cholesterol are due simply to the presence of a high proportion of animal fats in the foods that are eaten. Diets rich in beef, pork, lamb, eggs, and whole milk, butter, or cream will contribute to the elevation of cholesterol above normal limits.

Still another factor which is known to add to the risk of coronary damage is *cigarette smoking*. It has been found that persons who smoke from 10 to 20 cigarettes or more per day are three times as likely to suffer from coronary disease as non-smokers. There are at least two ways in which cigarette smoking affects the heart adversely. For one thing, the nicotine in cigarettes causes the heart to beat faster, and the end arteries to constrict, which in turn raises the blood pressure. Thus the work load of the heart is increased, and along with it the need for oxygen. Also, the smoke which the cigarette user inhales reduces the air-exchange capacity of the lungs, and thus their ability to provide oxygenated blood for the heart muscle. It is easy to see that the person who smokes cigarettes is forcing his heart to perform under two additional handicaps: he is increasing its work load, while at the same time he is reducing the oxygen supply it must have to perform that work. Since pipe and cigar smokers usually do not inhale, they incur much less risk as a group than cigarette smokers (though according to some authorities, their risk is still greater than for those who do not smoke at all). But the effects of smoking can be reversed, and it has been shown that the risk for cigarette smokers who quit is about the same as that for non-smokers.

In addition to these known physiological risk factors, a

number of others are strongly suspected by most physicians to be related to coronary disease. One of these is *family history*. Several studies have shown that coronary artery disease occurs with greater frequency among persons whose brothers, sisters, parents, or children suffer from the disease than among those whose family members are unaffected. In addition, such contributory conditions as hypertension, hypercholesterolemia, and diabetes are known to be influenced by heredity. What influence heredity may have on heart disease apart from these contributory diseases is not yet known, but some authorities believe the risk of developing coronary disease is increased by a factor of 1.7 for those persons who have a family history of the disease.

Another often suspected factor in coronary disease is *obesity*, which may be defined as 10 to 20% above one's ideal body weight. The overweight person places an extra work load on his or her heart. Further, obesity is often associated with elevated blood pressure, diabetes, and high cholesterol. However, it is not clear whether obesity operates as an independent risk factor or whether it affects the heart indirectly through these associated conditions. Some physicians believe that obesity is no more common among persons with coronary disease than it is among the rest of the population. In any event, whether or not obesity contributes directly to heart disease, doctors are unanimous in advising that it is a condition to be avoided or corrected by anyone who wishes to guard his health.

Physical inactivity is still another factor which is often thought to be implicated in coronary disease. A number of studies have produced data which strongly suggest that persons whose jobs require regular physical activity are less likely to have heart attacks than those in sedentary occupations. In one study, Irishmen living in Boston were found to have more heart attacks than their blood brothers living in Ireland. The one factor which was thought to account for this difference was that the American brothers rode to work by car or subway, whereas those in Ireland walked or rode bicycles. A similar study found more coronary disease among male clerical workers in Oslo than among their brothers who were farm laborers. Still a third study compared London bus drivers and conductors. The conductors, who had continually to climb the stairs of the double-deck buses, had less coronary disease than the less active drivers. Other researchers, however, pointed out that this study failed to consider the role of emotional stress, which would presumably be greater for the drivers. Indeed, when the drivers and conductors were divided into those who worked in the congested inner city and those who traveled the suburban routes, it was found that suburban *drivers* had less coronary disease than inner-city *conductors!*

Some physicians believe that exercise may lead to the development of collateral channels in the coronary artery system and thus provide alternate routes for the blood if main arteries are occluded. Although as yet there is no proof that this is true, doctors are nevertheless unanimous in recommending *moderate* and *regular* exercise as an important general health measure. It helps to reduce many of the other known or suspected risk factors—such as blood pressure, heart rate, blood fats, body weight—and generally leads to a better feeling tone both physically and emotionally.

Another factor suspected in the causation of heart disease is a *diet high in fats and/or sugars.* Laboratory experiments have demonstrated that cholesterol plaques can be produced in animals by feeding them high-cholesterol diets, and that these plaques can be reduced and even made to disappear through the restoration of normal nutrition. As mentioned above, high levels of fat in the bloodstream may result from hereditary metabolic disease as well as from diet. In a study conducted in Seattle, about 20% of heart attack patients were found to have one of several types of inherited hyperlipidemia. However, in a significant proportion of the patients in this study, elevated lipid levels were due to diet rather than heredity. It would appear that persons wishing to prevent the early onset of coronary disease should avoid excess fats and sugars in their diet, and should restrict their over-all calorie intake so as not to gain weight, or, if they are already overweight, to lose weight. Lean meats, fish, and fowl; non-fat milk; and fruits and vegetables should be the staples in such a diet. In general, "fad" diets should be avoided. Readers who wish more information on diets should consult the "Suggestions for Further Reading" at the end of this book. Persons who intend to pursue an intensive program of weight-reduction should consult their physician first.

Social and Emotional Risk Factors

But the physiological risk factors in coronary disease are only part of the picture. For years many experienced physicians have believed that social and emotional factors are involved in the onset of heart disease, even though the scientific evidence for this belief was relatively weak. As far back as the early 1940s, researchers were beginning to uncover evidence that certain kinds of emotional tension can contribute to coronary occlusion. Flanders Dunbar, an early psychosomatic investigator, sketched a personality profile of the coronary patient which consisted of compulsive striving, self-discipline, hard work, and a strong desire to excel.

Somewhat later, another researcher, Stewart Wolf, was to coin the term "Sisyphus reaction" to describe a common emotional pattern found among heart attack victims. Sisyphus may be remembered as a figure in Greek myth who because of his offense against the gods was condemned to roll a great stone to the top of a mountain, only to have it roll back down again immediately, so that the process had to be repeated endlessly. Dr. Wolf used the figure of Sisyphus to describe the person who strives with intense effort against great odds, but who gains little sense of reward or accomplishment from his labor. This pattern, identified through a psychiatric interview, was found to be significant in a study comparing heart patients and healthy persons. The research team was able to predict with an accuracy much greater than chance which individuals in the study were most likely to suffer a future heart attack and/or sudden death.

A number of studies have uncovered evidence of a rather non-specific kind of emotional stress or tension among persons with coronary disease. One group of investigators found that men who had suffered a myocardial infarction exhibited the following signs of tension significantly more often than a comparable group of healthy men of the same age: high divorce rate, loneliness, excessive work hours (25% worked more than 70 hours per week), heavy fluid consumption (including coffee, tea, and milk!), night eating, sleep disturbance, nervousness, anxiety, and depression. It was also noted, however, that one third of the heart attack victims did *not* fit this pattern of tense, restless behavior. Therefore, the researchers suggested, the absence of stress is no guarantee against coronary disease.

Two Swedish medical researchers compared 106 male heart attack victims with a group of healthy men of the same age. The heart patients tended to have four or more older brothers or sisters, to have completed little formal education, to have been rejected for military service, and to work 60 hours or more per week more often than the healthy group. It would appear from this that they were persons who had "come from behind" and had had to struggle against a handicap. The investigators recorded their impression that the younger heart attack victims, especially, had been "non-adapters" long before the onset of their coronary disease. The same team sought to determine whether such physiological risk factors as smoking, high blood pressure, and high cholesterol are influenced by social factors, or whether the two operate independently. Though they found some evidence for interaction between the two kinds of risks, they concluded that for the most part psychological and social risk factors operate independently of the physiological ones.

Another team of investigators has tried to establish a relationship between significant life changes and the onset of coronary disease. A Swedish study found that men who had suffered sudden death following a heart attack had experienced a marked increase in the frequency or intensity of such changes during the six months preceding their death. These included such experiences as the death or serious illness of a family member, divorce or separation from spouse, financial or business reverses, arrest or imprisonment, moving to a new home, losing a job or being promoted to a new position (not all the changes were painful or undesirable events). Similar results were obtained from a study of men who had survived a heart attack, whereas a small group of healthy friends of these surviving patients showed no significant increase in life changes for the three years preceding the study.

Still more evidence that social and emotional forces play an important role in heart disease comes from an intensive investigation of a single American community. Roseto, Pennsylvania, a town of 1,700 persons which was settled by Italian immigrants in 1882, was found to have a surprisingly low rate of heart disease. Over a twelve-year period, the death rate from myocardial infarction in Roseto was less than half that of several neighboring communities; moreover, none of the conventional marks of coronary heart disease was found among persons under 55 years of age in Roseto. Yet when compared to their neighbors in two nearby communities, the residents of Roseto did not appear to possess any advantage with respect to the well-known physiological risk factors. Though they had less diabetes than their neighbors, they were more likely to be overweight. Their serum cholesterol was about the same as that of persons in the nearby towns. Although their casual blood pressure was somewhat higher, they had less documented hypertension than their neighbors. Their diet was just as high in calories and animal fats as that of their neighbors; smoking was as common in Roseto as in the other two communities; nor did the Rosetans engage in any more vigorous exercise than those who lived near them.

What explains the extraordinary protection that citizens of this small town seem to enjoy against coronary heart disease? The answer to that question may come from an in-depth sociological study which showed Roseto to be an unusually cohesive and mutually supportive community where persons have strong family ties. Life in Roseto was described as family-centered, with no poverty and little crime. The research team was impressed by the high degree of mutual support and understanding which they found in the social climate of this unusual community, where residents could always find help from their neighbors in time of trouble. Those Rosetans who did succumb to early heart disease appeared to be persons who for one reason or another had become alienated from the mainstream of their culture. The inference from this study is that consistent social and emotional support affords significant protection against coronary disease.

Among the researchers who have studied the relationship between heart disease and personality type most thoroughly are two San Francisco cardiologists, Meyer Friedman and Ray H. Rosenman. In 1974 they published an eminently readable summary of their findings for the non-professional, *Type A Behavior and Your Heart*. During the early years of their practice, Drs. Friedman and Rosenman concentrated on such well-known physiological risk factors as cholesterol, diet, exercise, and smoking. But as time passed they became dissatisfied with this approach. In one study they compared the diet of a group of prominent businessmen with that of their wives to test the hypothesis that, since American women develop coronary disease much less frequently than men, the wives would show much less fat in their diet than their husbands. They were surprised to discover the same percentage of fat in the diet of both men and women. One of the wives in the study, however, was not surprised at all. "It's not what our husbands eat that is causing them to have heart attacks," she declared. "It's the stress they encounter in their work." Later they conducted an opinion survey of 150 businessmen. More than two thirds believed that the outstanding characteristic of friends who had suffered heart attacks was "excessive competitive drive and meeting deadlines." A majority of 100 practicing internists who participated in a similar survey agreed in describing their own coronary patients. Doctors Friedman and Rosenman next turned to a study of their own patients. Among them they found three outstanding personality characteristics: a habitual sense of urgency with respect to time; a very high degree of competitiveness; and a hostility that was easily aroused. Thus was born their concept of Type A Behavior.

Still unanswered, however, was the question how such a personality pattern could bring on coronary disease. Some light on this question has been shed by research on the relationship between behavior and cholesterol, which shows that the level of cholesterol in the bloodstream may vary directly with the intensity of the Type A pattern. In one study a group of accountants was followed from January through June, with cholesterol measured at frequent intervals through blood samples. As the April 15 federal tax deadline approached, the accountants' cholesterol rose sharply, only to drop again in May and June. During this time their diet, exercise and smoking habits remained the same. In another study, 80 men who were judged to exhibit a high degree of Type A behavior were compared with a group of 80 men in whom this pattern was absent (Type B). The Type A men had significantly higher levels of cholesterol in their blood than their Type B counterparts, though their diet and exercise habits were almost identical. Moreover, though all these men were supposedly healthy, it was found that more than one fourth of the Type A's *already* had coronary heart disease —a rate seven times as high as among the men who were Type B. Findings from these studies were further supported by laboratory studies. When the hypothalamus in the brain of a laboratory rat is damaged, this normally docile animal becomes vicious, hostile, and competitive—a close parallel to Type A behavior among humans. At the same time, rats upon which this operation has been performed also exhibit a marked elevation in their serum cholesterol.

In order further to test the significance of their findings,

Doctors Friedman and Rosenman undertook a prospective study of 3,500 healthy men, to see whether their concept of Type A behavior could be used to predict in advance which persons in this group would develop coronary disease. In a period of more than 10 years, over 250 men developed coronary heart disease. Neither diet nor exercise data was found to have much predictive value. The most significant factor— other than blood pressure, diabetes, smoking, and levels of fat in the blood—was the Type A pattern. Further, those persons in the study who did have high blood pressure, diabetes, hereditary hypercholesterolemia, or who smoked more than 15 cigarettes per day, were no more susceptible to coronary disease—and usually less so—than those who exhibited only the Type A pattern.

These researchers are convinced that one of the most important factors in the development of coronary disease is a lifestyle committed to a chronic, incessant, aggressive struggle to achieve more and more in less and less time. The Type A person is in constant conflict with the clock, the calendar, and the date book—and with his co-workers, friends, and family as well. He habitually sets his deadlines too early, and schedules too many events and projects for the time available to complete them. Often he appears to be absorbed in money, but this is secondary to his larger obsession with numbers of all kinds. He is an incorrigible scorekeeper, whether the score is figured in yearly income, number of scholarly articles published, percent of court cases won, or the yield of bushels per acre on the land he farms. The Type A person may appear to be extremely self-confident; in reality, he is haunted by the spectre of failure. And failure to him does not necessarily mean losing his job or experiencing financial reverses. It may mean simply doing no better this year than last, for what especially concerns the Type A person is his *rate* of progress, in whatever terms he may choose to measure it.

Little has been said about the person who is Type B, who is portrayed as the exact opposite of the Type A: free of habitual time urgency, excessive competitive drive, and easily aroused hostility. Since the A-pattern is found more frequently among men in America, the Type B person is more likely to be a woman. This person is less likely to have high blood pressure or to smoke heavily than the Type A individual. He or she is not necessarily any less intelligent, ambitious, or successful than his or her Type A counterpart, even though the stereotype of the successful executive in America incorporates large chunks of Type A behavior. Although the person who is Type B is by no means immune to coronary disease, he or she is much less likely to develop it during mid-life than persons of the opposite type. Therefore the Type B person is likely to live longer than his or her counterpart. Most important, this person will live with a greater sense of contentment and satisfaction than someone who is a confirmed Type A, since he or she is not struggling constantly to accomplish more than was achieved last year, last month, or last week. He or she can relax and enjoy the intrinsic rewards of work, play, art, nature, friendship, or love without feeling anxious or guilty about wasting time or worrying about deadlines still unmet.

Two points are important enough to be restated. First, not all Type A persons will succumb to coronary disease; neither will all Type B individuals escape it. The risk factors are probabilities derived from the observation of large groups of people. But probabilities are not certainties, and the experience of a particular individual may run counter to all statistical projections. Second, what differentiates those individuals whose behavior is thought to be "coronary prone" from others does not seem to be hard work as such, but rather a state of mind characterized by unremitting insecurity, anxiety, and hostility. The Type B personality may work just as long a day and with as much effort as the person who is Type A. However, the former is not striving anxiously and continually to outdo himself or his co-worker. Therefore he can enjoy the work itself, or the results of his work, or both.

Reducing the Risks

What we can do to prevent coronary heart disease should be clear from the preceding discussion. Anything that will counteract the various known or suspected risk factors should also reduce the likelihood of coronary disease appearing in the middle decades of life. What does this mean, specifically?

1. Any diseases which make one more vulnerable to coronary disease—such as high blood pressure, diabetes, or hereditary hypercholesterolemia—should be promptly identified and treated by a physician. The value of periodic checkups and, if needed, of regular follow-up treatment is evident. Although this sounds simple, not all people will find it easy to follow this guideline. Those with high blood pressure are not apt to notice any symptoms with their condition, and it may be difficult to persuade them that they must take medicine daily for the rest of their lives for a "disease" that only appears as a statistic in their medical record, at least for the time being. Those who suffer from diabetes and hereditary hypercholesterolemia may have to live with diet restrictions that seem irksome to them, or that deprive them of foods that have important personal meanings for them.

2. Those who smoke cigarettes should kick the habit as soon as possible. If they cannot quit smoking entirely, they should cut their use of cigarettes to less than a pack—better, to 10 or less!—per day. Those who have not taken up the habit and those who have previously given it up should resist the pressure to begin smoking.

3. All of us should strive to follow a diet that is relatively low in animal fats, and low enough in calories to prevent our becoming overweight; or if we are obese, to lose weight. Those who must struggle constantly to control their weight will find *The American Heart Association Cookbook* a valuable ally in their daily battle (see "Suggestions for Further Reading").

4. Regular and moderate exercise is an important facet of

any program for the prevention of coronary disease. Both adjectives need to be stressed. Experienced physicians are unanimous in warning that strenuous exercise is dangerous for persons 35 and older unless they have recently undergone a stress test for the presence of coronary disease. The stress test is a tracing of the electrical current produced by the heart recorded while the subject is exercising on a treadmill. The usual electrocardiogram, taken while one is lying down, will show damage that has already occurred to the heart muscle, but ordinarily will not reveal blockage in the coronary arteries which may cause future damage. Though not infallible, the stress or exercise EKG may disclose the presence of such blockages *before* they result in angina pectoris or myocardial infarction.

During a recent year, approximately 200,000 men who had never shown any symptoms of coronary heart disease died suddenly, more than one third of them during or shortly following vigorous activity. Further, the benefits of an exercise program are soon lost unless it is maintained regularly. The "weekend athlete" who lives a sedentary life Monday through Friday, but occasionally goes out to play handball or tennis singles after days or even weeks of inactivity is exposing himself to needless and foolish risk. Much wiser is the person who finds time each day in his schedule for walking, swimming, bicycle riding, or other moderate activity.

The person who consistently follows the four guidelines given above will do much to minimize the major physiological risk factors which contribute to coronary heart disease. For the man or woman of religious faith, these rules are more than just prudent preventive medicine; they are an application of the ethic of stewardship to our own bodiliness. Judaism and Christianity teach that human beings are responsible to the Creator-spirit for the continued care and use of all that has been given them.

> Do you not know that your body is a temple of
> the Holy Spirit within you, which you have from

God? You are not your own; you were bought
with a price. So glorify God in your body.

1 CORINTHIANS 6:19

Following sound principles of preventive health becomes not
just good common sense with an eye to survival, but a part
of the discipline through which men and women of faith
offer their lives daily in gratitude and service to the Giver
of Life.

But what about the social and emotional risk factors? Can
these be changed? Is it possible significantly to reduce mental
stress and tension, to reshape our behavior, rebuild our personality pattern? Surely it is too much to expect that we
could completely eliminate stress and tension from our lives.
Few of us are fortunate enough to live in a town like Roseto,
and even if we could identify and locate more such favored
communities, the sudden influx of population would no doubt
spoil them! Though some of us experience more stability in
our lives than others, none of us can protect ourselves fully
against events and circumstances which may alter our lives
profoundly. Serious illness in the family, unemployment or
business reverses, marital and family crises come our way in
spite of the most carefully laid plans. Even if we could protect
ourselves from such changes, the question remains whether it
would be desirable to do so. For many of us, a life protected
against change and the personal and social stress it may bring
would soon prove dreadfully boring.

The story of a husband and wife from a midwestern city
is suggestive. They had enjoyed their summer vacations at a
resort community in the Rocky Mountains so much that
when time came for them to retire they bought a home there.
After one year, they sold it and moved back to the midwest.
In the summer the resort community bustled with activity
from the influx of summer visitors, but when fall came, all
but a relatively few permanent residents left. During the
long winter the couple found little to break the monotony
and isolation except for the daily round of the rural mail

carrier! They discovered that some novelty and stimulation were essential to their well-being, that life could be *too* calm and uneventful, and that without some change and challenge the days could become dull and hum-drum. Many of us, I suspect, would react in a similar fashion. Perhaps we need to recognize that some degree of social change—and the stress that may accompany it—is not only inescapable but even necessary. At any rate, for better or worse it seems to be part of the fabric of our existence and we may as well learn to make the best of it.

Granted that we cannot eliminate all external stress from our lives, what about that which we generate for ourselves, internally? Can the Sisyphus reaction or Type A behavior be altered in persons for whom it has become a habitual pattern of existence? There is no point in denying that basic and fundamental changes in attitude or behavior are extremely difficult to achieve for people in the fourth or fifth decades of life. Those of us who have spent more than half a lifetime rehearsing our anxiety, depression, or hostility may have to struggle for the remainder of our lives to conquer these tendencies in the same way that a recovered alcoholic has to resume his battle for sobriety anew each morning. Yet, though such change is difficult and costly to achieve, no one can declare it impossible. If an alcoholic can conquer his drinking problem and go on to become governor of his state and later a highly respected U.S. Senator (as did Harold Hughes of Iowa), who can say it is impossible for a confirmed Type A person to give up his habitual restlessness, competitiveness, and hostility in favor of a more relaxed and cooperative style of life? Drs. Friedman and Rosenman are firmly convinced that it *is* possible for the Type A person to change and they offer a number of specific guidelines and exercises for anyone who wants to alter his style of life. Their confidence is supported by the experience of many such persons who have changed *following* a serious heart attack. One of these was the Kentucky poet-novelist Jesse Stuart who suffered a nearly fatal attack in the middle 1950s, and later published a book telling the story of his recovery. The title is significant: *The Year of My Rebirth.*

Religious teaching also strongly affirms the possibility of significant change in persons' loyalties, attitudes, and characteristic behavior. A familiar scene from the New Testament describes an encounter between Jesus and a prominent member of the religious community named Nicodemus. Jesus tells Nicodemus, "Truly, truly, I say to you, unless one is born anew, he cannot see the kingdom of God." But Nicodemus is sceptical that such fundamental and far-reaching change is possible. "How can a man be born when he is old?" he asks. "Can he enter a second time into his mother's womb and be born?" Is it really possible for someone in the midst of life to start all over again, as though at the beginning? To reshape and redirect the course of his life? To become a new person? Jesus' reply affirms both the possibility and the mystery of such a basic redirection of life. "The wind blows where it wills, and you hear the sound of it, but you do not know whence it comes or whither it goes; so it is with every one who is born of the Spirit" (John 3:3, 4, 8).

How is such change possible? In the Christian faith it is seen to come not primarily through drills and exercises, but rather as a result of the interplay between *grace* and *faith*— that is, through a trustful human response to a loving initiative of the Divine. An anonymous poet of the turn of the century said it well:

> I sought the Lord, and afterward I knew
> He moved my soul to seek Him, seeking me;
> It was not I that found, O Saviour true,
>   No, I was found of Thee.

> I find, I walk, I love, but, oh, the whole
> Of love is but my answer, Lord, to Thee!
> For Thou wert long beforehand with my soul;
>   Always Thou lovedst me.

The transformation of our attitudes and behavior occurs

indirectly, as a by-product of a new relationship with God. A changed life-style is not so much the end result of strenuous effort and goal-directed striving as it is "the fruit of the Spirit." But notice the nature of this fruit: "love, joy, peace, patience, kindness, goodness, faithfulness, gentleness, self-control" (Galatians 5:25). How different these qualities are from the characteristics of the coronary-prone personality: anxious, restless, impatient, always in a hurry, habitually engaged in competition, easily provoked to anger. Could it be that one of the best defenses against premature heart disease is a relationship of genuine trust in God?

Perhaps after all it is not so much a matter of trying to change ourselves, but of allowing ourselves to *be changed*. If so, the most significant contribution we can make to the process of change may be simply to wait expectantly for, and upon, God.

> Wait for the Lord;
> be strong, and let your heart take courage;
> yea, wait for the Lord!
>
> PSALM 27:14

> ... they who wait for the Lord shall renew their strength,
> they shall mount up with wings like eagles,
> they shall run and not be weary,
> they shall walk and not faint.
>
> ISAIAH 40:31

Is there anything we can do beyond waiting, trusting, hoping? Can our own efforts contribute to the process of change? I believe they can, and I want to close this chapter by suggesting three things which we can begin to do to support these processes.

1. We can begin now to re-examine, re-evaluate, and re-assess our lives. In doing so, we will need to look not only at our successes and failures, but, more important, at our goals as well. We need to ask ourselves not only, "What have I accomplished up till now?" but also, "What do I *really want*

to accomplish this year . . . during the next five years . . . before I die? Are my goals worthwhile? Will attaining them bring me lasting satisfaction and a sense of significance?" We will need to make some estimate not just of the quantity of our achievements but of their quality as well. We must learn to pay attention not simply to such outward signs of fulfillment as income, status, approval of our superiors, and respect of our peers, but to the inward marks as well—peace, self-respect, and a sense of fulfillment.

2. We can begin to practice the virtues of receiving as well as giving, relaxing as much as striving, listening as well as speaking, accepting as much as seeking to control. We can begin to remind ourselves that *being* and *becoming* are at least as important as *doing;* and that both are far more important than *having* and *possessing.*

3. We can begin to view life as an assignment in cooperation rather than competition. When even the simplest day-to-day activities become a contest to see who is the winner, persons become walled off from each other in closets of loneliness. When cooperation replaces competition as the guiding principle of relationships, persons experience themselves as part of the network of mutual caring and support. The parable is an old one but bears repeating: A man dreamed that he was being taken on a journey through hell and heaven. In hell he saw people sitting across from each other at long banquet tables loaded with food, but no one was eating. Each person had a long spoon chained to his or her wrist; the handle extended so far that no one could get the spoon from his plate to his lips. And so they sat, starving at a banquet. To the dreamer's surprise, the sight in heaven was almost the same—the long banquet tables loaded with food, the long spoons chained to the wrists. But here everyone was joyfully eating; each person was feeding the neighbor sitting on the opposite side of the table. Cooperation and caring for others can make the difference between a famine and a feast, a hell and a heaven.

The person who can begin to act upon the guidelines developed in this chapter will not only minimize the risk of incurring coronary heart disease, but will also maximize the quality of his or her life in the present, physically, emotionally, socially, and spiritually.

3

Recovering from a Heart Attack

Kenneth Madison is a highly successful, 46-year-old attorney. Until recently, his busy law practice occupied not only his weekdays, but many of his evenings and weekends as well. Work had gradually crowded recreation and relaxation out of his schedule. Golf, tennis, and swimming, all of which he had once enjoyed, became increasingly rare pleasures, as did camping trips which the entire family used to take. Ken had promised himself numerous times that he would quit smoking, but so far he had found it impossible to give up cigarettes for more than a few days. To light up and inhale was one of the few ways he could still find to relax for a moment in the midst of his crowded schedule.

Three days ago, Ken was hurrying back to his office after having lunch with several business associates. Although he felt some unfamiliar pain and fullness in his chest, he dismissed it as indigestion. But after he returned to his office, the pain returned, this time more severe than before. He began to sweat profusely, he felt nauseous, and he experienced difficulty getting his breath. The thought flashed through his mind, "It can't be a heart attack! I haven't got time to be sick now!" But as the pain became more and more intense and radiated from his chest to his shoulders, arms and jaw, he knew he had to do something. He called his secretary, who saw at a glance that her employer was desperately ill. By the time an ambulance had arrived, Ken was gasping for breath and his pain had become almost unbearable. The emergency medical team administered oxygen and a sedative which helped to relieve his pain.

The next thing Ken remembers after the arrival of the ambulance is waking up in the Coronary Care Unit of the hospital with an IV tube in his arm and electrical leads on his chest connecting him to the heart monitor at the head of his bed. His pain had subsided, but he was very weak and extremely tired. The nursing staff was quiet, competent, and reassuring. He needed only the look on his wife's face, however, to confirm the fact that the unthinkable had indeed happened—he had suffered a heart attack.

Kenneth Madison has just survived the first critical stage of a myocardial infarction. He is fortunate in having had emergency medical care available during this crisis, and in having been able to reach a hospital with a well-equipped and well-staffed coronary care unit. Now he moves into the stages of recovery from his heart attack. He will remain in the CCU for several days until the physician in charge is sure that the immediate threat to his life is past. This will complete the first stage of the recovery process for Ken. When he no longer needs the heart monitor he will be moved to another area of the hospital. The length of his hospital stay may vary from ten days to several weeks, depending on the extent and severity of heart muscle damage resulting from his infarction. Eventually he will move into stage three, convalescence at home, where he will gradually resume normal activities of daily life. The fourth and final stage in his recovery will come when, with his doctor's permission, he returns to work, perhaps for only a few hours a day at first, but later, as he is able, to full time employment.

Let us consider the emotional and spiritual aspects of each of these four stages in turn.

Denial, Dependence, and Despondency

One might expect that the predominant emotion with which Ken Madison has to deal is *fear*. After all, his life has been and still is very much at risk. Few of us have not known friends or co-workers who were less fortunate than Ken and who failed to survive the initial crisis of their infarction. We know that the mortality rate during this period is high. Yet, Ken does not remember feeling afraid, either before the ambulance arrived, or when he regained consciousness in the CCU. Distressed at the thought of leaving piles of unfinished work on his desk, yes; but not terrified at the prospect of imminent death. In this respect he is not unusual. Rather, his experience seems remarkably similar to that of many other heart patients. Compare, for example, the following two cases reported by psychiatrists Thomas P. Hackett and Ned H. Cassem.

A physician in his fifties felt severe chest pain while waiting for a plane. Since it passed quickly he thought no more of it until after takeoff, when the pain returned, along with shortness of breath. He told the stewardess he was having a heart attack and asked for oxygen. The pilot radioed ahead for an ambulance to meet the plane. By the time they had landed, his pain was intense and he realized fully the meaning of his symptoms. Yet at no time during this crisis did he experience the fear of death. It was only later in the recovery process, as he thought about returning to work, that he began to become concerned about how much longer he might have to live.

Another patient, a man in his twenties, developed severe chest pain while moving freight. Since he was physically exhausted from going to school full time and working in addition, his heart attack came as no surprise to him. He asked a friend to drive him to the hospital and then called his wife to tell her. On the way to the hospital he had to fight back the desire to drive by his home for a last look at his two children. Feeling close to passing out, he considered asking his friend to give him mouth-to-mouth resuscitation, but decided against it. When he arrived at the hospital he was near shock, and aware that every breath might be his last. Yet he felt no fear of death, nor could he explain his lack of fear.

Doctors Hackett and Cassem have conducted several psychiatric studies of persons in coronary care units as a result of myocardial infarction. Their studies suggest that conscious fear may be the exception rather than the rule among heart attack victims, at least in the beginning. The great majority of patients they interviewed used denial as a way of coping with the threat of their illness. Some patients rationalized their fears, others simply avoided talking or thinking about their illness, and still others concentrated on minor worries or discomforts (such as hemorrhoids) to the exclusion of the major threat to their life itself. Some patients, whom the researchers described as *major deniers,* insisted that they experienced no anxiety whatsoever as a result of their illness and hospitalization; others, described as *partial deniers,* admitted some concern, but tended to minimize their fears. In one of their early studies, 12 out of 19 patients interviewed were classified as major deniers, 6 as partial deniers, and only 1 as a non-denier! A later study of 50 patients identified 20 major deniers, 26 partial deniers, and only 4 minimal deniers. Significantly, those patients who were able to use denial effectively appeared to the researchers to benefit from it.

Although conscious fear of death does not seem to play a major role among heart attack victims at the time of the initial crisis, that does not mean that the experience does not have its full share of painful emotions. In one of the studies of Drs. Hackett and Cassem, 40 out of 50 patients interviewed were judged to be *anxious,* and 29 showed signs of *depression.* None was so depressed as to be incapacitated, however. (For the distinction between *fear* and *anxiety* see Chapter 6, page 98.) *Anger* was expressed by 11 patients, though it was usually directed against fate or circumstances rather than against persons. Eight of the 50 patients were noted to be *restless, agitated,* and *hyperactive.*[1]

Nevertheless anyone who talks with heart attack victims in the hospital learns of positive feelings that frequently accompany their anxiety, depression, and anger. "They sure take good care of you here. . . . Boy, these nurses really know their business. . . . They see everything that happens on that monitor out there at the desk." Such comments reflect the deep gratitude and trust the patients feel for the high quality of medical and emotional support they receive, as well as the relief and reassurance that go with the experience of being cared for sensitively and with competence. Also, one wonders whether there may not be something gratifying for such persons in having to let go, surrender, and give up attempts at controlling (often over-controlling) their own lives or the lives of others.

A close friend remarked that his awakening in the hospital several days after a sudden infarct that almost claimed his life was "the most blissful feeling" he had ever experienced. Although he declined to elaborate on this remark, I am inclined to speculate on its meaning. I knew him prior to his heart attack as a restless, conscientious person who was overburdened with heavy professional responsibility. Was his awakening in the CCU "blissful" because now, for the first time in years, there was nothing he *had* to do? All his responsibilities, all his obligations were now in abeyance. All he could do now was to lie back and allow himself to be waited on. Having devoted himself for years to the urgent needs of others, he could now allow others to devote themselves to his needs. His situation was not unlike that of an infant who is the center of his family's attention, who has only to screw up his face as though he were going to cry to mobilize their total concern and solicitude. It would

be wrong to label such a feeling "infantile regression," as
though it represented some deep-lying pathology. All of us,
I suspect, need the experience of being cared for, of depending on and being nurtured by others, not just at the beginning of life but periodically throughout the whole of life.
Many people, however, cannot accept their own need temporarily to be dependent, passive, and receptive. Their identity and sense of self-worth demand that they always assume
an active, giving, productive role. For such persons, a serious
illness may provide the only circumstance in which they can
surrender to the need to be cared for. The crisis of a heart
attack may give them a deeply gratifying and refreshing
opportunity to give up their over-investment in activity, in
control, and in shouldering responsibility on behalf of others.

The enforced inactivity which is imposed on the heart
patient may also have other, less desirable consequences. Prevented by his illness from using the most familiar and effec-
tive means of coping with anxiety, the heart attack victim
may find that the passive role he is forced to adopt with its
many physical restrictions leads to feelings of helplessness,
vulnerability, and depression. The novelist Jesse Stuart describes such feelings as he lay in the hospital after a near-fatal
heart attack. He felt as though he were in his grave, so weak
and powerless that he didn't even want to move. As his mind
regained its capacity to function and he became aware of his
situation, he was so depressed that he believes he might have
committed suicide if the means had been available. He felt as
though something had gone terribly wrong with him; something had taken place which he was powerless to change.
Lying under an oxygen tent, he grew weary of the familiar
faces that surrounded him—his wife, his doctor, his nurses.
Though he realized they were struggling to save his life, he
felt unable to participate in or be grateful for their efforts.
It seemed to him that it would be better if they simply allowed him to die and thus be free of what felt like a hopeless
situation.[2]

First Steps

In a few days when he no longer requires such intensive life-sustaining measures, Ken Madison will be transferred from the coronary care unit to another hospital area. In a moderate sized hospital this may be a general medical nursing unit; in a larger hospital it could be a specialized area devoted to the care of cardiac patients. His reactions to this move will probably be mixed. On the one hand he will be relieved and grateful to be leaving the CCU, because it means his condition is improving. Yet he may feel some twinges of apprehension. What will happen if his heart begins to act up now that he is no longer connected to the monitor? Will the nursing staff become aware of his difficulty in time to give him the immediate attention he received during the past several days? And what about the new staff he has to get to know? He has become quite close to the personnel of the CCU; he has learned to depend on them and has absolute confidence in them. Will his new nurses give him the same kind of sensitive and competent care he has come to expect during his stay on the coronary care unit? He can only wait and see.

Now begins stage two of the recovery process for Ken. Little by little the restrictions on his physical activity will be lifted, and he will become less directly dependent on the nursing staff for care. At first he may be permitted to sit in a chair beside the bed for brief periods; then to stand with help, then to take a few steps around the bed in his room. He will be surprised and perhaps dismayed at how difficult these simple tasks have become, and at how much strength he has lost as a result of his heart attack. As the days pass he will be allowed to use the bathroom by himself, and encouraged to walk in the hall—with help at first, and later on his own—for gradually increasing distances. Before he leaves the hospital, Ken will probably be able to shave himself, take a tub bath, and walk up and down a flight of stairs.

He may be placed on a carefully graded program of exercise

under the supervision of his physician. In some hospitals a physiotherapist would be assigned to work with him in his exercise program. The kind and amount of activity he is permitted will depend largely on the extent and severity of damage to his heart muscle.

How well Ken is finally able to adapt socially and emotionally to his heart attack, however, will depend on more than his physical status. Researchers have found that there is no necessary connection between the physical severity of a heart attack and the victim's ability to cope with the resulting problems. Some patients with little physical damage have severe social problems, while others with considerably more damage make a good adaptation.[3] Ken's successful rehabilitation from his infarction will depend on many factors. These include not only the physical capacity of his heart, but also his personality, motivation, and previous experience in meeting crises; the attitude of his family; the quality of his relationship with his physician; the availability of other well-trained members of the rehabilitation team; and his religious or spiritual orientation as well.

The Family Responds

At this point we need to pause and look at what is happening to the Madison family while Ken is in the hospital. They are deeply affected by his illness and hospitalization. Sometimes we overlook the family in the process of medical treatment. In a time of acute crisis, such as a heart attack, enormous attention is focused on the sick individual and his or her bodily processes. Modern medicine has made great progress by isolating and identifying pathology, by locating the specific organ or tissue that is diseased. In this process we can easily lose sight of the fact that disease always affects the entire person—not just the liver, or the lungs, or the lymphatic system. Further, it affects the person not just as an isolated individual, but in the total network of his or her relationships; disease has an impact upon the entire social system of which the sick person is a part. Unfortunately, comparatively little research has been devoted to this dimension of illness.

Some useful insights can be gained however from a study conducted by a British social worker and psychiatrist, who interviewed 65 wives of men admitted to a coronary care unit for their first myocardial infarction, both during the hospitalization and at intervals of 3, 6, and 12 months following his discharge.[4] All the wives reported considerable distress at first, with the suddenness of their husband's illness bringing numbness and panic. Many had a feeling of unreality in the beginning. Feelings of loss because of the damage they felt their husbands had sustained were also quite common, as were fears of recurrence, disability, and death. The investigators found considerable guilt and self-reproach among the wives concerning their husbands' illness, with many blaming themselves for making too many demands on their spouses, for not taking them more seriously, or for failing to protect them from overwork. Depression and anxiety were also frequently experienced, the most common symptoms of which were disturbances of sleep and appetite. Twenty-eight of the women showed more severe grief reactions; these occurred more often among the younger wives (those under 45 years of age) and among those who had a previous history of emotional disturbance. Psychosomatic symptoms related to the husband's illness—such as headaches, stomach aches, faintness, chest pains, and palpitations—were reported by more than one-fourth of the wives.

Generally the women felt relieved when their husbands were able to return home, yet for some of them this was a very trying period. Twenty-five women reported anxiety, depression, tension, and difficulty sleeping at this time, for which they gave two major reasons. The first was their sense of loss in having a weak and "damaged" husband, and their fear that the illness would recur. How much activity the husband could safely tolerate was a source of great concern to

many, as was also the recurrence of chest pain and the consequent anxiety over whether to call the doctor. It is not surprising that some of the wives reacted to their anxiety by
becoming over-protective and trying to shield their husbands
from any stress or upset. The second reason the women gave
for their anxiety was the changed attitude and behavior of
their husbands. A number of the men seemed to their wives
to be either more dependent than before their heart attack, or
more irritable, or both. No matter how hard they tried to do
the right thing, some of the wives found they could not please
their partners. If the wife appeared concerned and protective,
the husband resented it; if she tried to be firm, she was seen
as cold and unfeeling. In a few cases the husbands actually
felt better after their infarction than they had during the
year before; and the wives of these seven patients were among
the least anxious when interviewed three months after
discharge.

One year after the onset of the illness, 26 wives felt their
husbands had made a good recovery, and judged that their
own feelings and their marital relationship were as good as
they had been before the illness. Another 23 wives were still
experiencing some anxiety and apprehension about their husbands, but their emotional disturbance was not great. The
remaining 16 women were still experiencing emotional disturbance severe enough to interfere with their own lives and
the lives of their families. In half of these families, however,
the husbands had not made a good physical recovery; four
had died, and three were disabled by their illness. Thus, only
12% of the wives failed to adapt when their husband's physical recovery was good. Further, only 10 women whose husbands had made a satisfactory recovery a year later reported
that their marital relationship had deteriorated during the
period of the illness. The husbands in these families were anxious, irritable, and demanding, and the wives tended to feel
guilty, to suppress their anger, and to overprotect their mates.

To sum up, the year following the heart attack was a difficult time for this group of wives; yet most of them were

able to make a fairly good recovery from the emotional and social crisis of their husband's heart attack.

Further light on the experience of the family of the heart patient comes from author Jacqueline Lair, who gives a vivid description of her reactions upon being told by a friend that her 36-year-old husband, Jess, had just suffered a heart attack in his advertising office.[5] Her first response was one of shock and disbelief: her husband couldn't have had a heart attack . . . he was only 36 . . . besides a heart attack might mean death, and Jess couldn't die . . . she needed him and loved him too much! At first she could not even bring herself to use the words "heart attack," much less "death." Yet in the midst of shock she was able to function physically and mentally and to deal with numerous immediate, practical problems. Though her heart was pounding, her mouth was dry, and she was short of breath, she was able to make decisions about how the children were to be cared for, who would drive their two cars home, and what to do about Jess's advertising business.

But she found herself dreading to see her husband. When she arrived at the hospital, accompanied by the friend who had brought the news of Jess's attack, she was unable immediately to face her husband. She had to stop and make one more phone call to give herself time to deal with the fear of seeing him. When she did get to see Jess, he looked strange and alien to her, with his ashen-gray skin, the oxygen mask over his face, and the intravenous tube in his arm. It was a relief when the nurse asked her to step out of the room so he could have his shot. Jackie also found herself reaching out for and accepting help from others at this time. She phoned a close friend simply to tell her what had happened, and asked her to inform their neighbors and their parish priest. She was able to ask some other friends to look after the advertising business temporarily. And she found comfort and reassurance in the crowd of healthy persons who gathered in the hospital waiting room to support her and Jess.

She describes still other feelings as well. One of them is *guilt*. Her mind rehearsed all the ways in which she might have been responsible for Jess's heart attack. She asked herself why she hadn't been more help to him, why she had been so impatient with him, why she had made so many demands upon him. She wondered why she had let him buy an expensive house in such an expensive suburb, or why she had allowed him to give her the sports car he had known she wanted. Along with the guilt she also had many feelings of *anger* toward Jess. Why was it that he always had to do everything the hard way, why couldn't he learn to relax and take life at a more sensible pace? (From both his own and his wife's account, Jess Lair appears to have been a classic Type A personality!) *Hope* is still another emotion that Jackie Lair experienced during this crisis. Her hope was mobilized in part by the ministry of their parish priest. Though she had not been devout in the observance of her faith for some years, Jackie found herself comforted by the familiar rite of extreme unction which the priest administered to Jess in the hospital, and this rite awakened her hope that Jess might survive.

Not just Jackie, but the entire family was affected by Jess's illness. She describes the loneliness at the dinner table without father present. The two oldest girls went on with their school work and social activities, but carefully avoided talking about their father. The nine-year-old son assumed his father's role as head of the household, sitting in his dad's chair at the table and getting up at 6:00 A.M. to shovel snow off the driveway. Their three-year-old became an inveterate thumbsucker and suffered speech and learning difficulties for the next several years, while the youngest child, at 18 months, responded to the tension in the home by clinging tightly to his mother.

When Jess returned from the hospital, Jackie felt great fear and uncertainty. Would he get along all right? How should she treat him? How much exertion could he stand? What kind of meals should she prepare for him? What if he were to have another heart attack? Suppose he should *die*—perhaps even in bed, by her side? She describes their first sexual experience after his illness, fearful, yet urgent with mutual need.

Finally, Jackie Lair discusses the changes that had to be made in their harried, hurried, and costly life-style. Together they decided to sell their expensive house in the suburbs, her sports car, and the advertising business. They found an inexpensive farmhouse to rent, moved to the country, and prepared for Jess to go back to the university to prepare for a career as a college teacher.

We can assume, then, that Ken Madison's wife and children are undergoing a very stressful time as a result of his heart attack. They are no doubt very anxious and uncertain about the outcome of this illness, for they know that it is life-threatening. Even when the immediate crisis is past and it appears that Ken will survive his infarction, they may still wonder whether their husband/father will be able to return to his normal life-style. Moreover, they are separated from him as a result of the illness; even though Susan, his wife, and the two older children can visit him in the hospital, they are very conscious that they are *visitors*. The hospital is not home, it is alien territory. Expressions of affection must be tempered in order not to upset Ken, and also because there is another patient who shares the same room, and privacy is difficult to achieve. Important conversations have to be interrupted because of routine hospital procedures. Finally, since life must go on for the Madison family, someone else has to take over the role that Ken played in the family. Decisions which would have been shared by husband and wife — such as whether thirteen-year-old Judy is mature enough for a boy-girl party—have to be made by Susan alone. Such household chores as mowing the lawn and washing the car have been taken over by fifteen-year-old Tom without his Dad's supervision as in the past. The family must learn temporarily to function without a key member on whom they have depended. Later on, when Ken is able to assume a more active role, this whole process will have to be reversed, and a place found for father once again.

Coming Home

The day that he returns home from the hospital will be a gratifying one for Ken Madison and for his family. It will be reassuring to know that he is making satisfactory progress and that his damaged heart muscle is beginning to heal. Ken himself may feel like a prisoner newly released from captivity. Yet both he and his family are apt to feel some apprehension and uneasiness as well. He is now considerably farther from immediate medical help than he was while in the hospital. How much does he dare to attempt? If symptoms recur— such as palpitations, tachycardia, or chest pain—how soon should he call the doctor? He doesn't want to appear over-anxious, but he is understandably fearful of another episode like this last one. His mind is running over with questions: How long will it be before he is able to go back to work? Will he ever be able to resume his former schedule? How much exercise can he tolerate? Will he be able once again to play golf and tennis, or go backpacking in the mountains? When will the doctor give permission for him to drive the car? And what about sex? When will it be safe for him to make love again with Susan? When the time comes, will his body cooperate? Right now even a little physical activity leaves him tired and weak.

(Although cases of myocardial infarction and even death following sexual intercourse have occasionally been reported, few physicians would enjoin a celibate life on most of their married heart patients. The energy expended during the sexual act by middle-aged, married adults has been estimated as comparable to that of climbing two flights of stairs. By using common sense and some restraint, most heart patients will be able to resume a satisfactory sexual life with their spouse. However, some drugs commonly prescribed for heart patients may affect their sexual function. Also, certain circumstances make the sexual act more than normally stressful and thus involve added risk for the person with heart disease. Among these are excessive drinking, having just eaten a large meal, and engaging in extramarital intercourse, especially if the partner is much younger and excessively vigorous. Heart patients and their spouses should ask their individual physician if they have questions about the appropriateness of sexual activity.[6])

With all of the uncertainty and apprehension that fills his mind, it would be easy for Ken to become overly-cautious and overly-dependent. His family members are eager to wait on him—why not let them take care of him? He might understandably choose to play it safe and avoid all possible risks. But this attitude could end in his becoming a cardiac cripple, a person needlessly disabled not by his injured heart muscle but by his own fears and anxieties. A 60-year-old man gave up his job as a jewelry salesman at the suggestion of his physician after having two supposed heart attacks. However, careful examination in a cardiac rehabilitation clinic nine years later disclosd no evidence of heart disease, but did result in a diagnosis of arthritis of the cervical spine. Informed that his heart was all right and that he now could go back to work, the patient refused. However he continued to attend the arthritis clinic regularly and insisted that if it were not for his arthritis he would have returned to work long ago! [7]

On the other hand, Ken Madison might react just the opposite way. Instead of becoming over-concerned about his health, he could behave impulsively and recklessly. He might disregard the physician's instructions concerning exercise, diet, and work, and stubbornly refuse to recognize the real limits his injured heart has placed upon him. If this should happen, his family might try to assume the responsibility for enforcing the doctor's rules—a role in which they would be very likely to fail.

It is hoped that Ken will be able realistically to accept the limits that are necessary for him without giving up or becoming a permanent invalid. He will no doubt feel especially weak, dependent and vulnerable at first, but this feeling should diminish as his physical recovery proceeds and his strength and vitality return. He may at times react irritably to his family's well-meaning attempts to assist him. After all, he does resent his weakness and his need to be helped, even though he recognizes it as real. He may also resent their health and vitality, so much in contrast to his own present condition. It would be surprising if there were not days when Ken feels depressed during this period of convalescence at home, for his diet is restricted (low salt, low cholesterol), his activities are limited, and he gets bored watching game shows and soap operas on television. He feels deprived of many things that made his life pleasant and comfortable before the heart attack —his cigarettes, his pre-dinner cocktail, an occasional Saturday golf game; but most of all, his work. Though he looks forward to regaining some of these pleasures in the future (minus the cigarettes), it seems to him that recovery is taking a very long time. Nevertheless, with the realistic hope that life will not always be like it is now, and with the patience of an understanding family, Ken should be able to make it through this stage of recovery to the final phase, his return to work.

And Back to Work

Ken is fortunate that his work is not unduly taxing physically. When his recovery process is complete, he will be able to return to his law practice, although he may have to modify his schedule. Evenings and weekends will have to be times of rest and relaxation for him instead of opportunities for going back to the office to catch up. He may need to limit his practice by accepting fewer new clients, or by specializing in certain types of cases only. At all events he must overcome the Sisyphus complex discussed in Chapter 2. He must make time in his life for activities that renew his body, mind, and spirit —for an occasional play or concert, a good book, moderate and regular exercise, an evening of conversation with friends, relaxing outings with his family, and participation in his church as well.

If Ken's work were more strenuous physically, or if his heart damage were more severe, it might be necessary for him to consider a change of vocation. This would require an assessment of both the job—its physical and psychological requirements and its consequences for the worker—and of Ken's own health, skills, and motivation. Then it would be necessary to match him with a job within his physical and emotional capacity. This might be done by comparing the known energy costs of his job-related tasks with the functional capacity of his heart.

In some cases the patient and job are matched by placing the person in either an actual or simulated work situation and monitoring his heart functions over a period of several hours. In addition to the physician, both the social worker and the vocational counselor may play an important role in this process. Heart patients who require retraining for a different job may be able to qualify for assistance from their state Division of Vocational Rehabilitation; and those who are completely disabled by their disease are likely to be eligible for Social Security and perhaps other benefits as well.

We should not suppose the physical consequences of a heart attack are the sole determinant of the person's ability to make a satisfactory adaptation to work, however. A study by Gelfand and associates compared heart patients who made a good vocational adjustment with those who made a poor one. The two groups did not differ medically or vocationally, but they did differ on social and psychiatric measures. Those who adapted poorly (were unable to work, worked below their capacity, or were trying to work beyond their capacity) reacted to their heart disease with overconcern, with denial, or with exaggerated adherence to the initial limitations imposed upon their activity. They appeared to be passive, dependent, and vulnerable to stress. Those who adapted well tended to have obsessive-compulsive personality traits, and were more stable and dependable than their less successful counterparts.[8]

Grief, Growth, and Grace

What spiritual tasks and challenges face Ken Madison as he recovers from a heart attack?

One is the task of learning to live in a more receptive mode. Like many of us, Ken has lived his life in the active mode, as a doer. We cannot know the extent to which this life-style may have contributed to his heart attack; in fact, not all physicians agree on the significance of personality and behavior patterns in the development of coronary disease. Nevertheless from a religious perspective it is clear that Ken has allowed his life to become unbalanced. He has overinvested himself in his profession, and he has tended to neglect his family. To be sure, he has not ceased to care for them or be responsible for them. Indeed, his evenings and weekends at the office were "for their sake," to enable him to provide them with the security and comforts of a large, well-furnished home in an upper-middle class neighborhood with excellent schools, a savings fund for the children's college education, and adequate insurance for emergencies. But in giving them all these things, Ken has unintentionally withheld from them a more important gift—himself, his time, his attention, his personal interest. What is more, in the all-absorbing task of providing for his family he has largely forgotten how to *enjoy* them. The first task that faces him now is to allow *them* to give to *him*, to give him their care, their affection, their solicitude, and then in return to begin to give them himself.

Ken has majored in managing and controlling events and circumstances for most of his life. He has always been competitive—in the classroom, on the athletic field, and in his law practices. This competitive drive made him a high achiever. But now he must learn to relax, to rest, to surrender in trust to other persons and to forces which he cannot control, but which will nevertheless sustain him if he will allow them to do so. Those forces include the marvelous recuperative powers of his own body, the medical expertise of doctors and nurses, the love of his family and friends, the beauties of the natural world, and the spiritual power of faith and hope. What Ken must do is to begin to open his life to what theologians call *grace*.

In the Bible, the word "grace" is derived from the word for "gift." It points to the gift-like character of all existence. For Ken Madison, as for many of us, life has been regarded as a prize rather than a gift, a prize to be won by intense struggle and disciplined effort. "The race is to the swift . . . The early bird gets the worm . . . Only the strong survive." Ken must learn that these are at the most only half-truths, that they are dangerously distorted guidelines for living. His first spiritual challenge is to realize that life is indeed a gift, to be received from beyond himself each day with gratitude, to be celebrated with joy, and to be shared with love. Orville Kelly, a cancer patient who became nationally known as the founder of the organization Make Today Count, tells of receiving a letter from a woman who had read about his work in the newspaper. She realized in reading the article that she had grown up in the same house where he now lived, and she wanted to know if the lilac bush still bloomed beside the living room window. "I didn't even know there was a lilac bush there," says Orville Kelly, "but I know it now, and I know when it blooms."

To learn to receive and enjoy his life as a gift from beyond himself—this is the first spiritual challenge which Ken Madison's heart attack sets before him. The second is to reassess and reexamine his life, his values, his priorities. What is most important to him? What does he believe in most deeply? How does he want to be remembered, by his wife, his children, his friends and co-workers? What changes will have to be made in his life if it is to reflect these fundamental values? Jess Lair relates that in the first few days following his heart attack he decided that he would never again do something he didn't deeply believe in. This resulted in his selling his home and business and in returning to school to prepare at age 36 for a completely new career.[9] Novelist Jesse Stuart describes the year following his heart attack as the year of his *rebirth*.[10] Although Ken Madison may not make any dramatic outward changes in his pattern of life, he is challenged by his illness to re-think his reasons for *everything* he does, to see whether they are consistent with his most fundamental concerns and loyalties.

Above all, Ken's illness presents him with the opportunity to *grieve* and *grow*. He must grieve because he has lost a part of himself—that strong, hard-driving, competitive person who could take his vital energy for granted because it seemed inexhaustible, to whom sickness and death were words that applied only to other people. His life has been permanently altered because of his face-to-face encounter with death; his diet, his work, his recreation, the attitudes of his family, and his expectations for the future are all different because of his heart attack. Yet he need not be overcome by this loss. Through it he may also grow in his understanding of the true purpose of his life, in his enjoyment of the simple pleasures of each day, in his appreciation of the worth of others, and in his trust in and commitment to God. As this growth takes place, he may experience the lasting significance of these words from the New Testament:

> We are afflicted in every way, but not crushed; perplexed, but not driven to despair; persecuted, but not forsaken; struck down, but not destroyed . . . So we do not lose heart. Though our outer nature is wasting away, our inner nature is being renewed every day.
>
> 2 CORINTHIANS 4:8-9, 16

4

When the Doctor Recommends Surgery

One Woman's Operation

Vivian Hellstrom is a 67-year-old widow who lives by herself in a small midwestern town. Her husband died eleven years ago. Two years ago, Mrs. Hellstrom retired from her job as bookkeeper at a lumber yard. Her three grown children, all married, and her seven grandchildren live in Kansas City, Minneapolis, and Seattle.

Mrs. Hellstrom had always been an active person. Before her husband died she worked with him in the frozen-food locker. After his death she sold the business but needed some additional income. Since she felt at loose ends being unemployed, she took a job at the lumber yard. She has always taken pleasure in her large lawn and garden, which she cared for herself until recently. She has also been active in church and community affairs, a tireless volunteer worker and committee chairman for all kinds of worthy causes. A vigorous and independent woman, her visits to her children have usually been brief because "there's so much I need to do at home."

But for more than a year now Mrs. Hellstrom has not felt like her old self. When cold weather set in a year ago last fall she began to have difficulty getting her breath. As the fall turned into winter, she found herself becoming unusually tired on her daily walk downtown to the post office. She began to notice chest pains when she engaged in any unusually vigorous activity, such as shoveling the snow off her front sidewalk. For a while she put off seeing her doctor, thinking she was just a bit run down and that it would surely pass. But as her tiredness increased and her bouts of chest pain became more frequent, she knew she ought to have a checkup.

Her doctor's verdict after hearing her complaints and examining her was "angina pectoris." He explained to her that her chest pains and shortness of breath were caused by a constriction of her coronary arteries, and that they could be brought on by strenuous effort, excitement, emotional stress, cold weather—in short, anything that caused her heart to have to work harder and demand an increase in its blood supply. For a time, he treated her medically. However, as the months passed, it seemed that her spells came more frequently and with less provocation. Her doctor confirmed her suspicion that her disease was progressing and referred her to a large medical center for evaluation for possible cardiac surgery.

Mrs. Hellstrom had to wait several weeks for her appointment. When the time came, she was driven to the clinic by a friend. After a preliminary examination she was admitted to the hospital for further tests. Mrs. Hellstrom had never had such a thorough examination. Not just her heart but every part of her body was subjected to the most searching examination. There were countless questions, many blood samples, numerous X rays. She found herself describing her symptoms and their onset again and again. After several days of this, the doctor in charge asked her permission to perform a cardiac catherization. "We are sure now that you have no major health problems except for your heart," he told her. "But we need to know more about the nature and extent of your heart disease before we can determine whether you would benefit from cardiac surgery."

He went on to explain the procedure to her. "This is not a treatment for your disease, but a diagnostic process which will enable us to describe the condition of your heart more completely and precisely. It does carry a small risk, as do many other medical procedures, such as having your tonsils removed. However, the risk is slight, and your heart disease also carries some risk, especially if it is left untreated." He went on to explain that a long, thin, hollow plastic tube would be introduced into a blood vessel and carefully threaded through the vessel up into her heart, and that the tip of the tube would then be inserted into the coronary artery. Then a substance which is opaque to X rays would be injected into the tube and an X-ray picture taken as this substance passed through the coronary arteries. From the movement of the dye the doctor would be able to tell exactly where the blood flow is obstructed in her coronary arteries, and to what degree. Although she might have some mild temporary discomfort, the procedure should not be painful to her.

"Is this test really necessary, Doctor?" asked Mrs. Hellstrom. "After the examinations you've given me, I didn't suppose there could be anything you didn't already know about me!"

"Yes, it is necessary if we are to know whether or not you can be helped by surgery, Mrs. Hellstrom," the doctor replied. "Of course, you could go home now, and we could continue to treat your angina medically. But by your own report it seems to be getting more severe, and I gather you're not very happy with the restrictions your heart disease places on your activity. We think surgery might benefit you, but in order to be sure we have to be able to describe the nature and extent of your disease much more precisely. This test is the only way we can do that."

Mrs. Hellstrom decided to proceed with the catheterization. Though she was somewhat apprehensive, she had been reassured by the doctor's careful explanation of the procedure. Most of all she was anxious to know whether surgery might offer her relief from the narrow limits into which her life had been thrust by her coronary artery disease. "If I just have to sit around the house waiting to die, my life's not worth much," she declared to her friends.

The catheterization was accomplished smoothly. Mrs. Hellstrom was back in her room within a couple of hours, with instructions that she must lie quite still for the next four hours. Late that afternoon the cardiology team came to her room to discuss the results of the test with her. After studying her X rays carefully and weighing the alternatives, they recommended that she proceed with surgery. They made it clear, however, that the decision whether or not to have the operation was hers. If she chose to accept their recommendation, she would be placed on the schedule at the earliest time, probably three to four weeks hence. The staff would be happy to suggest to her the names of several other patients who had undergone a similar operation and who were willing to discuss their experience with others, in case she wished to consult with them in making up her mind.

In one sense Mrs. Hellstrom had already made her decision; she asked the doctors to place her on the surgery schedule as soon as possible. Yet she did accept the names of the other patients. The next morning she was discharged from the hospital and returned home to wait until the date for her surgery.

The next few weeks were difficult ones for Mrs. Hellstrom. She would have preferred to have the operation right away and to have it over with, instead of having to live in anticipation of it. Though she was eager for the benefits of the operation, she also found herself dreading the experience. One of the thoughts that came to her mind was that she might not survive the operation. She knew that there is some risk to life in all major surgery, and it seemed to her as though this operation, involving the central organ on which life depends, must be very "major" indeed! Though the doctors had assured her that the risk of dying in surgery was small, they would not deny that it was present. Another set of fears revolved around the pain she knew she would experience after surgery. Would she be strong enough to endure it without whining or complaining, without losing her dignity and composure? Still another concern was disfigurement. Although it was not a major worry, Mrs. Hellstrom did wonder how large the scars might be from her incisions, and whether they would be noticeable to other people. Most of all, perhaps, she worried about the outcome of the operation. Would it really help her as much as the doctors thought? Even they couldn't provide any guarantee of success. How terrible it would be, she thought, if she were to go through all of this and then find that she was no better than before. But she was reassured by her visits with two patients whose names the doctor had given her; both were pleased with the outcome of their operations and encouraged her to go ahead with her plans.

Mrs. Hellstrom made the time pass while waiting for her operation by tidying up her house. She was helped in this by the arrival of her youngest daughter from Seattle, with her four-year-old son. Since she would be unable to be present during her mother's surgery, she wanted to have this opportunity to visit her. The week with her daughter and grandson, whom she had not seen for more than a year, helped to keep Mrs. Hellstrom from becoming unduly preoccupied by anxiety over her surgery.

The day finally came for Mrs. Hellstrom to be admitted to the hospital. A bed had been reserved for her in the cardiac surgery unit. Her operation had been scheduled for early the following morning. It was a busy afternoon and evening— more X rays and blood tests ("What in the world do they do with all that blood?" she wondered), a brief visit from the surgical team, a conference with the anesthesiologist who would attend her during surgery. Then her son, daughter and son-in-law arrived to stay with her until she was out of the Intensive Care Unit. The hospital chaplain also dropped by late that afternoon. "Your pastor at home wrote us that you would be coming and asked that one of our staff call on you," he explained. He assured her that he would return as soon as she was alert after surgery, and that in the meantime he would visit her family while they waited for her. Before leaving, he offered prayer at her request. Finally, after visiting hours were over for the evening, the nurse came in to prep her for the operation.

The operation for which Mrs. Hellstrom was being prepared is known as an aorto-coronary artery bypass graft, a procedure which was recently developed and which is becoming more and more common in major medical centers for the treatment of coronary artery disease. In this operation, a vein is removed from the patient's own leg and is used to reroute the blood around the blocked portions of the coronary arteries. A portion of this vein is connected to the aorta at one end, and at the other to the blocked coronary artery below the site of the obstruction. The blood supply is thus restored to that portion of heart muscle which has been deprived by the blockage and the patient's anginal pains are relieved. Although Mrs. Hellstrom was to have only two grafts, more than five may be performed during a single such operation, depending on the extent of the patient's disease.

In this operation the heart-lung machine is used to maintain the patient's circulation during surgery. This machine, also known as the pump-oxygenator, was developed in the mid-1950s. It receives the patient's blood through tubes attached to the major vessels which return blood to the right side of the heart (the inferior and superior venae cavae); this blood is passed through a pump and oxygenating machine to clear it of carbon dioxide and replenish it with oxygen; then it is returned to the body through the aorta. Thus the pump takes over the function of both the heart and the lungs while the surgeon operates. Mrs. Hellstrom's surgery was possible only through the disciplined cooperation of a large number of people, including surgeons, cardiologists, anesthesiologists, operating room nurses, clinical laboratory technicians, a perfusion technologist (who operates the heart-lung machine), blood bank personnel, and her own family physician who referred her in the beginning for evaluation.

Mrs. Hellstrom awoke early on the morning of her operation. The sleeping medication prescribed for her had helped her to spend a reasonably restful night. Her son, daughter, and son-in-law arrived shortly after she awoke and she found their presence reassuring. Before long the nurse came with her preoperative injection, and she soon found herself becoming quite drowsy. By the time she kissed her children good-bye and was loaded on the surgery cart, she was even feeling slightly euphoric.

She can recall only fragments of the next twenty-four hours. She does remember opening her eyes at one point to find her daughter and son-in-law standing by her bed and asking them, "Why haven't they come for me yet?"

"Mother, it's all over," her daughter replied. "You've had your operation and the surgeon says you're doing fine. You're in the Intensive Care Unit now." She can also remember the nurses and doctors urging her frequently to breathe deeply and to cough. Although she found this quite painful, she did her best to cooperate, since it had been explained to her before surgery how important it was for her recovery to keep her lungs clear of mucus. As consciousness gradually returned, she became aware of the great many wires and tubes connected to various parts of her body. Since these had been described to her beforehand, she was not surprised or alarmed by them, but she was greatly relieved when the doctor was able to remove the endotracheal tube from her throat on the second day. As another item of equipment was disconnected every few hours, both her comfort and her appearance improved. Her family was surprised and delighted by the rapid change they could see taking place. It made their anxious day of waiting through her surgery abundantly worthwhile.

On the afternoon of the second day after surgery, Mrs. Hellstrom had improved enough to be transferred out of the Intensive Care Unit back to the postsurgical ward. Here she would begin her reentry into normal daily activities, first by sitting in a chair, eating solid food, using the bedside commode and then the bathroom, and walking, gradually increasing distances in the hall each day with the assistance of a nurse or physiotherapist. Rather to her surprise, she did not have as much pain as she had expected, but she did feel very weak and tired the first few days. As the days passed, however, she found her strength and vitality returning bit by bit. By the eighth day following her surgery, her doctor felt it would be all right for her to return home. Her sister planned to come and stay with her for the first couple of weeks. A return appointment was scheduled for her at the clinic a month later so the doctors could review and evaluate her progress. Mrs. Hellstrom felt glad to be going home, grateful for the skill and dedication of the hospital staff, and immensely relieved to have her operation over with and behind her.

Heart Surgery: An Overview

The advent of surgery on the human heart is relatively recent. As late as 1882 the great German surgeon Theodore Billroth warned his colleagues against ever attempting to suture this vital organ. Yet by the early years of the present century, surgeons were able to drain fluid from the pericardial sac, to repair stab wounds to the heart, and to remove cysts or tumors immediately around the heart. These, however, were operations on the *outside* of the heart, which could be performed while the heart was still beating. Operations on the *inside* of the heart were still some years in the future. A further step toward modern open-heart surgery came in the early 1930s, with the repair of patent ductus arteriosis by a Boston surgeon. This condition—in which the aorta and the pulmonary artery are connected by a small vessel which normally disappears shortly after birth—was repaired by clamping the connecting vessel at each end and then cutting it. Later, it was discovered that a stenotic mitral valve could be opened by the surgeon's inserting his finger through the heart wall and breaking open the scar tissue which held the leaves of the valve together. Although the tricuspid valve could be repaired in the same manner, the pulmonary and aortic valves were more difficult to reach and did not respond well to such approaches. All of these were essentially *closed heart* operations, performed while the heart was still carrying out its function of pumping blood throughout the body.

The development of *open-heart* surgery had to wait for the invention of the heart-lung machine described in the account of Mrs. Hellstrom's operation. This device, which became operational in the 1950s, permitted surgeons to stop the heart and get inside the chambers themselves to repair defects. At present a number of kinds of open-heart surgery are performed frequently in large hospitals. Diseased or damaged heart valves may be repaired, or even replaced entirely with artificial plastic valves, or with valves transplanted from the hearts of people who have died from other causes. Defects in the septum between the right and left pumping chambers may be closed by suturing or patching, as may also holes between the right and left receiving chambers. Narrowed pulmonary and aortic valves may be opened surgically, and complex congenital defects, such as tetralogy of Fallot, which involves both a defect in the wall between the ventricles and a narrowed pulmonary valve, can be corrected. The aorto-coronary artery bypass graft described earlier in this chapter is becoming an increasingly common procedure. And, of course, a number of heart transplants have been attempted in some centers.

This latter operation has not yet become a standard method of treatment, not because of any defect of surgical skill in implanting the heart, but rather because of the difficulty in solving the problem of rejection. When foreign matter of any kind is introduced into the body, its own defense system develops antibodies to protect it against the "invader." Unless the body's own defenses are suppressed, this process will result in such inflammation and damage to the tissues of the transplanted heart that it will eventually cease functioning. The production of antibodies can be decreased by the use of immuno-suppressive drugs; but if given in too great a quantity, these drugs reduce the body's needed resistance to infections. Hence, the great majority of the more than 200 persons who have undergone heart transplants have died either from cardiac rejection or from infection. Some researchers hope that in the not-too-distant future a mechanical device may be perfected which can be implanted within the body to replace the human heart.

The reader may wonder just how typical Mrs. Hellstrom's experience is. In many respects she appears to be an ideal case: her surgery was successful, her recovery was rapid and smooth, and she was able to handle the emotional stress associated with her surgery in a mature and constructive way. Needless to say, things do not go that smoothly for all persons who undergo open-heart surgery. In some cases the operation fails to bring the hoped-for improvement; in others, the recovery process involves complications and requires a more extended period of time. Occasionally the patient shows more signs of emotional disturbance than did Mrs. Hellstrom. Rarely, the patient may not survive the operation, or may die in the hospital. Nevertheless, I have seen many patients undergoing open-heart surgery whose hospital course was strikingly similar to that of Mrs. Hellstrom. Such a favorable outcome depends not only on the high degree of technical skill and sophistication of the surgical team, but also on careful screening and selection of patients for surgery by the medical staff, and on thorough preparation of the patient, mentally and emotionally as well as physically.

What about the thoughts and feelings of patients who undergo open-heart surgery? In my observation it is common for patients to have a certain amount of anxiety about this procedure ahead of time. According to a recent nursing study, the most frequently cited source of emotional disturbance in patients awaiting open-heart surgery was anticipation of what the future would hold. Included in this category were fears not only of death, pain, and helplessness, but numerous other concerns as well. Moreover, the patients in this group did not always show their anxiety openly. They communicated their uneasiness by direct speech a little less than half the time; by indirect conversational clues another third of the time; and the remainder of the time by nonverbal signs or body language.[11]

But anxiety and apprehension are only part of the story; along with them one discovers in these patients a considerable amount of hope and determination. The hope comes from their expectation of a better, fuller, more active and normal life. It is this hope, standing in contrast to the person's frustration and dissatisfaction with his or her present state of health, that produces a sense of determination and a willingness to undergo the risks, the pain, and the inconvenience associated with surgery. "I'm no good the way I am now, so I might as well have the operation. I've got a lot more to gain than I have to lose," or, "I don't have much choice; I can't go on the way I am now," are typical statements of persons who elect this type of treatment. Once they have decided to have the surgery, these persons are usually eager for it and may appear quite calm and cheerful when admitted to the hospital for their operation. They may feel little need to talk about their apprehension and anxiety, indeed they may minimize and even deny these feelings. One suspects that some patients do not welcome any conversation which might weaken their resolution to proceed with the surgery or which would raise doubts about whether they have chosen the wise course.

After the operation, one occasionally sees signs of transient depression in the heart surgery patient. On a number of occasions patients have said to me, about the third or fourth day following their surgery, "If I had known how hard this was going to be, I would never have let them do it." However, these same patients are likely to feel quite differently about their decision a few months later, provided the operation is successful. By this time they have begun to experience the benefits of restored health and renewed vitality; they are able once more to enjoy familiar activities, and to work productively. And in a number of instances I have known patients who submitted quite willingly to open-heart surgery a second time.

These impressions derived from my experience as a hospital chaplain are supported by a 1972 survey of nearly 800 persons who had undergone heart surgery. Although 71% reported that they were anxious before the operation, almost the same proportion described themselves as having been optimistic about the outcome of their surgery beforehand. For most of these patients the immediate postoperative period was very stressful; two-thirds stated that they experienced anxiety, depression, confusion, or feelings of unreality during this phase. Nevertheless, nearly all of the respondents (96%) said they were glad they had the operation. Substantial gains in physical ability were reported, with the typical patient's ability to climb stairs or walk long distances having doubled following surgery. Three-fourths of the group felt psychologically improved after surgery. The areas in which the greatest gains were reported were "pleasure in life" (79%), and "job performance" (76%). The area in which the fewest patients reported improvement was "sexual relations" (49%). Though many patients had made significant gains by six months following surgery, others took a year to realize the full benefits of the operation.[12]

Religious Resources for the Surgery Patient

What spiritual and religious factors support the person who must face open-heart surgery? What attitudes seem to aid recovery and healing?

One is the courage to face painful and unpleasant realities directly and realistically. The person contemplating heart surgery must be aware of a number of uncomfortable facts and possibilities. One is the fact of the disease itself, and its probable course if surgery is declined. Another is the risk to life involved in the operation. Still another is the physical and emotional distress that must be endured following the procedure. The possibility that the operation may not produce the hoped-for results is still another. Sometimes people whose lives are crippled by heart disease are so anxious for relief that they hear all the positive and hopeful things the cardiologist says about the proposed surgery, but screen out all the negative possibilities. Such people can become deeply disillusioned, depressed, and angry if their hopes are not fulfilled. It requires considerable spiritual strength to face such threats to one's being without taking refuge in comforting illusions or fantasies, and to make the decision for (or against) surgery in full awareness of *both* the benefits and the risks. It is not surprising then frequently to hear religious people confess, "If I hadn't known that God would be with me through it all, I could not have done it."

Another important attitude is the capacity to trust and depend on others to care for us and fulfill our needs. In the encounter groups which were so popular a few years ago, trust in one's fellow group members was sometimes expressed by allowing oneself to be led blindfolded around the room by another person; or by falling backwards freely and permitting oneself to be caught by others; or by letting oneself be picked up and carried on the shoulders of the entire group. But these exercises in trust are mere charades in comparison to the trust demanded of the patient facing heart surgery. Many writers comment on the symbolic significance of the heart. In everyday language as well as in classic literature it is much more than just a pumping mechanism; it stands for the whole person, indeed for life itself. When the patient allows the doctor to take his heart in his hands, even to open the heart and place his hands inside it, he is surrendering his very life into the surgeon's hands, both symbolically and literally. Frequently it is even necessary for the surgeon to stop the heart so as to have a more quiet operative field, and then to restart it again when the reconstructive work is finished. If we are unable to trust others, to allow ourselves for at least a brief time to become totally dependent on them, it will be extremely difficult for us to give ourselves up to the ministrations of the surgical team.

One may ask, is there any connection between this kind of trust and the trust in God that religious people call *faith?* I believe they are related, though I would caution that they are not identical. Those who profess no religious commitment may become very trusting patients; whereas others who find it difficult to give themselves up to the doctors' care may nevertheless be genuinely devout individuals. What is crucial, I believe, is the *capacity* for trust, whether in God or in other people. The person who has developed that capacity can direct his or her trust to an appropriate source of care, whether divine, human, or both. The believer knows that only God, the ground and source of all being, is worthy of total and unreserved trust. The faith believers place in their doctor is always, therefore, a limited and qualified trust. Yet people of faith also believe that God's will is always and in all ways directed toward the fulfillment of persons; therefore they believe that in giving themselves up to the care of a competent team of physicians they are at the same time placing themselves in the care of a loving God who uses the skill and dedication of the medical team to accomplish his purposes. The mother of a young boy who had been helped to survive massive burns once remarked, "I make no distinction between a medical miracle and a religious miracle." She knew that God is the ultimate source of all healing, though the means may include medicine, surgery, skilled nursing care, physical therapy, and many other instruments.

What has been said about the necessity of trust must be balanced by a third essential spiritual factor: the determination to cooperate to the fullest extent in the healing process. Patients undergoing open-heart surgery cannot take a completely passive, dependent role. Though they must be willing to allow others to wait on them and care for them, they also must be enlisted as active participants in the whole enterprise. This will become especially important in the postoperative phase, when they must learn to breathe deeply, to cough up phlegm from their lungs, and to exercise. Though these may be difficult and painful tasks for some patients, they are absolutely necessary. The goal of recovery can only be achieved through the combined efforts of the patient and the health care team. Indeed, the patient is an essential part of this team, without whom the team cannot function.

That patients sometimes do allow themselves to become too dependent on the hospital environment and personnel is suggested by a recent nursing study of persons who had undergone cardiac surgery. When interviewed five to six weeks following their discharge from the hospital, many of the patients were still reluctant to engage in a number of activities of which their doctors felt they were capable, such as climbing stairs, doing housework, shopping, light gardening, driving a car, or taking part in social and recreational activities. Walking was the most strenuous activity in which most of this group engaged. Generally the patients seemed to be more uncertain about what they could do following surgery than they had been prior to their operation. They had known their limitations before surgery; afterwards they seemed to feel anxious and insecure if they exceeded these old limits, even though these limits were no longer appropriate.[13]

Thus, if the goal of successful and full recovery is to be achieved for the cardiac surgery patient, the capacity to surrender and entrust oneself to the care of others must be combined with determination to be a full and active participant in the struggle for healing.

Finally, a fourth spiritual resource must be mentioned: faith in God as the one who will fulfill his purpose for our lives in spite of illness, disability, and even death itself. It is my conviction that God intends for every individual the fullest measure of health that can be achieved. I see God as unreservedly on the side of healing, and as an active participant in the struggle against pain, weakness, and incapacity. Hence I have no hesitation about praying with patients facing heart surgery for their recovery, for relief from pain and distress, for the renewal of their strength, and for their liberation from the crippling bonds of disease. I do not even feel it necessary to add the classic disclaimer, "if it be thy will," for I am sure this is God's will for humankind. Yet I also recognize that life is a precious but exceedingly fragile gift, hemmed in on every side by dark forces which limit, thwart, and distort it. And at the far horizon of every life looms the final mystery of death which none of us shall escape. Why a God who intends health and vitality for his creatures has placed us in such a flawed and threatening universe I cannot explain. But I am sure that his purpose for us will not be defeated by these dark realities.

A congregation which I once served had experienced a series of tragic deaths among its members. As an expression of their faith, which had been severely shaken by these losses, the people incorporated into their Sunday service a closing response to the benediction, sung by the whole congregation in words from a hymn by John Greenleaf Whittier:

> I know not what the future hath
> Of marvel or surprise,
> Assured alone that life and death
> God's mercy underlies.

The faith that our life *and* our death, our joy *and* our pain are encompassed by a divine purpose that is both gracious and invincible can enable the person who must submit to heart surgery to face dark and threatening circumstances realistically, to entrust his life to the care of a competent surgical team, and to join with them actively and with determination in the mutual struggle for healing.

5

Children as Patients

As we noted in Chapter 1, about one in every 1,000 babies is born with an abnormality of the heart. Many of these children will need an operation, some during the first few months of life, others at a later time. This chapter is intended to help parents whose child must undergo cardiac surgery.

This situation is sure to awaken many painful feelings in parents. Some mothers and fathers may feel ashamed or guilty, as though they had somehow failed their child by bringing him or her into the world with a defective heart. Others may feel angry and resentful that their child should have to suffer. Their anger may be directed toward God, or toward medical personnel who have to administer painful procedures in the hospital, or even toward one another, as though each blames the other for the child's condition. And, of course, there is a high degree of anxiety present in the parents over the successful outcome of the child's operation, and his consequent survival and recovery. Parents must first recognize and deal with their *own* painful feelings before they can help their child deal with his anxieties about hospitalization and surgery. Although they may often be able to do this without outside help, a third person such as a social worker, chaplain, or family counselor may occasionally provide invaluable assistance in understanding, accepting, and expressing these feelings.

Preparing a Child for an Operation

The impact of illness and hospitalization on the child will vary depending on the child's age at the time surgery is undertaken. Very small infants of six months and under have little understanding of their external environment and are not greatly distressed by the absence of parents so long as their basic physical and emotional needs are met dependably. Children of school age are old enough to understand something of the nature of their illness and the reasons for their hospitalization, and can tolerate parental absence for periods of time, though they may feel sad, lonely, and afraid. The experience is probably most difficult for children who are six months to five or six years of age. It is especially difficult for those one- and two-year-olds who are very much aware of their environment but have not yet learned how to communicate through speech. Separation from their parents is very threatening and disturbing to these youngsters. The very young child cannot know that his mother will return when she leaves, or even that she still exists when she is out of his sight and hearing. The British psychiatrist John Bowlby has shown convincingly that very young children separated from their parents for periods of several weeks go through a process that is almost identical to the grief adults experience when they lose a loved one through death. Thus it is extremely important that younger children be separated from their parents as little as possible, or that if parents are unavailable, a consistent and adequate parent-substitute be provided.

For this reason an increasing number of hospitals make provision for a parent to "room-in" with a preschool child and to participate in the child's care while in the hospital. Most hospitals which do not provide for rooming-in have adopted lengthy and flexible visiting periods for parents of small children. Of course it is sometimes impossible for a parent to stay at the hospital with the child, whether because of employment, illness, or responsibility for the care of other children. In such cases as these a parent-substitute, such as a trusted aunt or grandparent, is much to be desired.

After age four, children can begin to grasp the fact that though their parents leave, they will return later. However, these children need much reassurance that their parents still love them, that they will return to visit them at a definite time, and that they will be going home from the hospital when they have recovered from their surgery. Familiar objects from home may help to reassure a child—a doll or teddy bear, a favorite blanket, familiar books or records. One of the ways in which children may respond to the threatening aspects of separation is by regressing to an earlier stage of development, such as talking baby talk, wetting or soiling themselves, or becoming irritable, demanding, or whining.

In addition to the anxiety they experience over separation, children have many other painful feelings related to hospitalization and surgery. Illness and medical treatment are frequently seen by children as punishment. A youngster suffering from pneumonia understood the medical reasons for his hospital stay, but also insisted that he was sick because God was punishing him. When asked how this could be, he explained that he had taken ill after playing outside in the snow without his overshoes for a long afternoon, and that his illness was God's punishment for having disobeyed his mother's instructions! Many workers with children therefore advise parents to explain carefully to their child that his heart condition is not his fault, nor is anyone else to blame for it. Children are also apt to feel angry, particularly over painful medical procedures, over examinations which violate their sense of modesty or need for privacy, and over restrictions on their activity which threaten their newly developed and hard-won independence. They may not be able to express this anger directly at the persons who elicit it, for they are likely to view doctors and nurses as very powerful adults who can do anything they please to a child's body, and thus fear retaliation if their rage is expressed. However, anger may often be revealed in play situations, depicted in pictures or stories, or acted out in games. It should not be stifled but allowed to find its needed and proper means of expression.

Children also have many fears, some realistic and some based on misconceptions or fantasies. Among these are fears of pain, disfigurement, disability, and death. For this reason it is important that children be prepared for their hospitalization and surgery by clear, simple and repeated explanations of what is to be done and why. These explanations should be suited to the child's level of intellectual and emotional development. Children should *never* be tricked or deceived into coming into a hospital, but should be told ahead of time that they will be going to the hospital, the reason why, and what they may expect to happen once they are there. Children seven years and older may be told several weeks in advance; children from four through six years, four to seven days ahead of time; and children two and three years, a few days in advance. For some children a drive by the hospital building may be a helpful part of the explanation. Parents whose own anxiety prevents them from preparing their child adequately for hospitalization undermine the child's sense of trust and security, and expose him to frightening misinformation and fantasies.

When it comes time to talk with the child about his operation, a doctor or nurse should offer a clear and simple explanation of what is to be done. For example, a five-year-old who is to have a septal defect repaired might be told: "Your heart is in the middle of your chest. It pumps the blood through your body to nourish you and help you grow and be strong. Your heart has a little hole in it that doesn't belong there. We don't know why it is there; it is something you were born with. But it makes more work for your heart, so the doctor is going to sew it up so it won't cause you any trouble." In addition, the location of the incision might be described for the child, as well as any tubes, IVs, catheters, and ECG monitor leads that he might have after surgery. He would be told that he must breathe deeply and cough up mucus, even though it is hard for him. The manner of coughing would also be demonstrated with the child.[14] In some hospitals dolls are used to inform the child about the procedure and to show him what he can expect afterwards. Sometimes children are also encouraged to play with safe items of equipment that are used in their treatment, such as tongue blades, surgical caps and gowns, a stethoscope, or syringes without needles, in order to help them feel more at home in the situation.

We cannot assume that explaining the operation to the child is all that is necessary. The child needs time to assimilate this information, to ask questions, and to act it out in play activities. The child may need to discuss the operation numerous times with adults and with other children in order to correct and clarify misunderstandings and to integrate his knowledge emotionally as well as intellectually. It is better for those preparing the child not to give unrealistic reassurance (e.g., "Don't be afraid, it won't hurt at all"), but to be honest about procedures that may be painful. Also it is very important that adults not discuss a child in his presence as though he were not there, or as though he were unable to understand what they are saying. Even children who have not yet learned to speak are much more aware of what is said about and to them than we usually realize. When children overhear themselves being talked about, but are unable to participate in the conversation, they may form distressing misconceptions, like the child whose doctor described him as having edema in his abdomen, and who later told his mother the doctor had said he had "a demon" in his tummy! Therefore, when the child is present, he should be *included* in the discussion as a full participant. Further, parents should seek to discover and correct any misinformation that the child may have acquired by providing frequent opportunities for him to ask questions, to describe his own understanding of the operation to them, and to express his feelings about it. Some authorities also stress that children need to be assured that no part of their body will be operated on other than the part described to them.

Children not only need adequate preparation before surgery, but also the opportunity to work through their feelings about the experience afterwards. Some children may act out the operation in play with another child or with dolls, perhaps assuming the role of doctor or nurse rather than patient. This may help the child achieve a sense of mastery over a situation in which he was relatively helpless. Other children may appear quite passive and even withdrawn, and may need the help of an adult to explain or act out their feelings about their experience. Still other children may react to surgery by becoming uncharacteristically aggressive and belligerent, and may need to have some limits set to this behavior. In any event, parents need to help "debrief" their child by encouraging him to talk out his feelings concerning his operation, or to act them out in play in nondestructive ways.

The remainder of this chapter examines the experience of two boys who underwent heart surgery. The accounts are based on interviews with the children and their parents one or two years following surgery.

Michael: "It's No Big Deal"

Michael is a bright, handsome and active nine-year-old who underwent surgery one year ago for a coarctation of the aorta (a constriction in the main vessel carrying blood from the heart). When Michael was an infant, a physician detected a heart murmur, and told the parents that although they need not be concerned at the time, they should have him checked later. Since he appeared healthy and developed normally, Michael's parents thought little more of this murmur until he was seven years old. At that time they noted that he seemed to be having some difficulty concentrating in school.

They asked a friend of theirs who was a senior medical student to examine him for possible neurological problems. In the course of the examination, the student discovered a difference in the blood pressure in Michael's right and left arms that led her to suspect he had a coarctation. This initial diagnosis was later confirmed by more exhaustive studies at a nearby medical center. Thus Michael and his parents knew that he would have to have an operation for about a year before he went into the hospital. How did he feel about this? "Nervous, but kind of excited, too." He was nervous because he anticipated that it would be a painful experience and he dreaded injections. But he was also excited because he looked upon it as a new adventure. ("They have TVs in the room that you can turn on from the bed.")

Michael entered the hospital for his catheterization in late March. He was prepared for this event ahead of time by his parents (his father worked in the hospital part-time and was familiar with the procedure) and also by members of the hospital staff. His memories of the procedure are somewhat hazy, since he was conscious but under sedation at the time. He remembers the doctors' introducing the catheter in the artery in his groin; he recalls hearing the staff talking, and talking to them; then at some point he believes he lost consciousness. When he returned to his room, he slept the rest of the afternoon and evening; the following day he went home. His parents' impressions of this event are more vivid than Michael's. His father was conscious of seeing the hospital from a very different perspective now that his son was a patient, and of feeling a closeness to other parents on the ward that he had not experienced before as a member of the staff. He was also aware of "the oppressive heaviness of time" during the long wait for the catheterization and the recovery period following it. Michael's mother, who was unfamiliar with the hospital environment, found herself quite distressed at being surrounded by the very serious medical, social and emotional problems of other children and families on the ward.

About three months later Michael entered the hospital for

his operation. This was explained to him by a pediatric nurse who brought with her a doll with tubes inserted into various parts of the anatomy to show Michael what it would be like when he awoke in the recovery room. What did he find difficult about the experience? "It wasn't so bad. The pain wasn't as bad as I expected. Things were just like they said they would be." He remembers being frightened only once: "When it was time for me to go to surgery, and they said, 'It's your turn now.' But then the ride on the cart to the operating room was kind of fun. When I got there the doctor asked me if I wanted the anesthetic through a little cut on my leg or if I wanted this bad smelling gas through a mask, and I said the mask. But I think I was asleep before they put it over my face." His parents recall that the removal of the drainage tube from his chest after surgery was momentarily quite painful; but Michael doesn't remember this as unusually distressing.

Michael remembers several good things about his stay in the hospital. "Everyone"—the doctors, nurses, and parents of the other children on the ward—"was very kind." He made several new friends among the youngsters his own age also having heart surgery at this time. "We had a contest to see who had the most stitches." He also remembers pulling "the plugs" (EKG monitor leads) to tease the nurses. "The first time they came running. After that they knew what was happening and didn't get so excited." His parents remember that on the day after his surgery, they found Michael sitting on the floor with his friends putting a puzzle together. His IV tube and monitor leads were connected, and he was perspiring from pain, but he was absorbed in the puzzle.

What was most difficult about the recovery period? For Michael, it was "learning to walk with all that stuff connected to me." But his parents have more somber memories of this period. When Michael's chest was opened during surgery, it was discovered that he had not *one,* but *two* constrictions in his aorta. His catheterization had failed to disclose this very uncommon circumstance, and the surgical team was unable to repair either defect at that time. They informed his parents that Michael would have to have another operation when he is eighteen, at which time both defects would be corrected. Thus the most difficult part of the experience for the parents was "finding out that he would have to have the operation all over again." Both they and Michael seem to have adapted to this prospect very well. Michael is an active, healthy-appearing child whose only handicap is that he can't run as fast as other children his age. He told me that he thought one of his doctors had said that his future growth might make surgery unnecessary, but his parents insist that no doctor has ever told them this, nor have they ever told Michael.

Michael's father regrets the way in which Michael was told that he would need another operation. The medical team came one day while Michael was still in the hospital to discuss the outcome of the operation with his father. Michael was apparently absorbed in a TV program and was not included in the conversation at first. As the discussion of his problem unfolded, it became apparent to the senior physician that Michael was actively listening to the conversation. He then turned to Michael and proceeded to explain the situation to him in simple terms. Michael does not appear to have been upset by this incident, but his father is chagrined that neither he nor the physicians took Michael into account at the beginning of the discussion. Two misconceptions had to be cleared up after Michael returned home from the hospital. At school, his gym teacher made a reference to Michael's "handicap." This troubled Michael, for he understood the word as a term for mental retardation, and his parents had to explain its broader meaning to him. Also, some time after his return home Michael's parents became aware of the fact that he thought his next operation might well be fatal, and that he had therefore only a limited number of years to live. They explained to him that the future operation would be no more dangerous than the previous one, and that, in fact, it might be less risky because of the improvements in heart surgery that could be expected during the next several years. Both matters appear to have been resolved successfully by these discussions.

Michael's parents did express some concern that many people outside the family seem overly solicitous about him, and enquire anxiously about his health as though he isn't normal. "They seem to want to make more of it than we do." Michael's response: "Yeah, they seem to think it's a big deal." The parent of a severely retarded teenager remarked on one occasion, "I couldn't cope with the problem you have."

If Michael had a chance to talk to another child who was facing heart surgery, what would he say? "Don't worry. It's not so bad. The pain isn't too bad, the food is pretty good, and you meet a lot of nice people." It is evident that Michael's surgery has left no permanent emotional scars, nor is he preoccupied with thoughts of his future hospitalization. During the year that has passed, the painful aspects of the experience have tended to fade from his memory, and are recalled more vividly by his parents than by Michael. At the time of the interview he appeared to be a very lively, engaging, and thoroughly normal nine-year-old.

Todd: "I Could Do It Again If I Had To"

Todd is now thirteen; he was eleven when he underwent surgery for an atrial septal defect (a hole in the wall which separates the right and left receiving chambers of the heart). When Todd was born, a pediatrician heard a heart murmur which he regarded as functional, but advised the parents that he should be checked later. Several years later another physician recommended that he be seen by a cardiologist. He was taken to a regional medical center some distance from his home, where surgery was recommended. However, Todd's parents were reluctant to submit him to an operation at this time. His father was in the last year of graduate school and it was apparent that they would be moving soon, but did not yet know where. More influential, however, was Todd's mother's experience. As an operating room nurse, she had worked with a well-known cardiac surgeon some years before, and was reluctant to expose her child at that time to what she regarded as a rather high risk of death. They decided to wait.

The next year they had Todd examined at the hospital connected with the university where his father was now teaching. The pediatric cardiologist there felt that since Todd was doing well they should simply wait and have him re-examined the following year. For several years they continued this, deciding each year not to proceed yet with surgery. Though Todd was the fastest runner in his class at school, and had won a president's physical fitness award, his heart appeared to have become significantly enlarged by the time he was eleven.

Early in June, Todd entered the hospital for his catheterization. His memories of this event are for the most part unremarkable, except for a rather lively party on the ward with two other youngsters scheduled for the same procedure the next day. He does recall the trip to the catheterization laboratory on a hospital cart; the doctor's inserting the catheter in his femoral artery; and the flushed sensation as the dye was injected. When the examination was finished, the doctor applied a pressure bandage to his leg. However, the first bandage came loose, there was a brief spurt of blood, and an annoyed doctor had to apply another bandage. Todd's parents report that when he returned to his room he experienced intermittent nausea and vomiting, but he does not remember this. He slept most of the rest of the afternoon and evening and went home the next day. He was permitted limited activity until the incision in his leg was fully healed a week later.

Todd's surgery was scheduled for late July. He was well prepared for his operation, first by his mother who was knowledgeable in this field and then by several members of the hospital staff who explained the procedures to him fully. Though he was unhappy at the loss of many of his summer and early fall activities because of the operation, he does not appear to have been fearful of the surgery beforehand. When

Todd awoke in the Intensive Care Unit, he was aware of a maze of wires and tubes connected to his body, but he does not remember feeling any pain. Only when it was necessary for the nurses to manipulate his chest tube to drain it fully did he have pain; then "it felt like they were pulling your insides out."

For Todd's mother and father this was an especially distressing time, however. Since he had felt well and appeared healthy, and did not want to have the operation, it had been difficult for them to make the decision to commit him to surgery. They discussed the matter with him and took his feelings into account, but accepted responsibility for the final decision themselves. To their first view after surgery, Todd appeared desperately ill, and they could not help but ask whether they had made the right decision. It was hard to credit the seeming nonchalance of Todd's surgeon: "Don't worry. He'll be sitting up watching cartoons by Saturday morning." (This was Wednesday afternoon; the surgeon's prediction proved to be accurate.)

Twenty-four hours after surgery Todd had improved so much and was becoming so alert and active that it was decided to transfer him from the ICU to the surgical cardiology ward. Here his progress continued to be rapid. He and the other children on the unit were allowed by the staff to be as active as they felt comfortable being. Soon Todd was walking the corridors pushing the stand with his IV bottle; taking the three-year-old across the hall for rides in a wheelchair; and as his doctor had predicted, watching cartoons on the TV in the day room. He was discharged six days following his operation, two days earlier than was expected.

Todd's activities were somewhat limited for the first three months at home; the doctor didn't want him engaging in any contact sports until his incisions were fully healed. After that time he was permitted to return to normal activity. In the two years since his operation his parents report that he has gained significantly in his energy level, endurance, appetite, and weight. His memories of his hospital experience are not particularly frightening or unpleasant. Some weeks after his discharge his father asked him if he thought he could do it over again if it were necessary. Todd answered that he could. If he had the opportunity to talk to another youngster facing a similar operation, he would tell him that he need not be afraid, that the experience is not painful. He showed no reluctance to reminisce with me about his time in the hospital.

While no attempt is being made to suggest that all children who undergo heart surgery have experiences like those of Michael and Todd, the accounts of their operations suggest that when children are carefully prepared for the experience ahead of time and receive adequate support and understanding from their parents and the hospital staff, their hospitalization and surgery need not be unduly distressing. Indeed, the child may often take it in stride as a difficult and challenging but growth-producing event.

6

Living with Heart Disease

A great deal of attention has been focused in recent years on the problems of the person who is terminally ill. During the past decade courses, seminars, workshops, books, journals, articles, films and TV programs have multiplied on the stages of terminal illness, the needs of the dying person, the reaction of family members, and how professionals can respond most helpfully to people faced with death. The disease most frequently mentioned in this discussion is cancer. Heart disease has often been overlooked in this connection because we do not usually think of heart disease as a "terminal illness." To be sure, many people do die of heart disease—more than from any other single cause. But many others survive heart attacks, and go on to live an active and productive life. One thinks of such persons as the late Lyndon B. Johnson, who recovered from a heart attack and went on to become majority leader of the U.S. Senate, then Vice-President, and finally President of the United States. Somehow the threat of death to the victim of heart disease seems less certain than to the person who has cancer. Yet the impact of heart disease may be every bit as great as that of cancer on the emotions, the personal relationships, the career, the financial security, even the life-expectancy of the person who is afflicted.

Although it may not be terminal, heart disease, like any other serious health problem, is apt to be life-threatening, life-shortening, and life-altering. In this chapter we shall consider the impact of such disease on the emotional and spiritual health of the affected person. Let us recall what was said in Chapter 1 about the meaning of the word "spiritual." The word here does not mean some inner part of the person which is relatively independent of the body or the mind. Rather it is used here to point to the wholeness and potential unity of the human being—body and mind, feelings and behavior, meanings and relationships.

Illness as a Spiritual Crisis

Any person who experiences a life-threatening, -altering, or -shortening illness such as that resulting from serious heart disease is faced with a number of threats to his or her spiritual integrity and well-being. As may be seen from Figure 1, the attacks come from at least four different quarters. The person is threatened first of all by *fear* and *anxiety*. Although we often use these words interchangeably, some writers make a useful distinction between them. Fear is the feeling we get when we face a known danger, such as a speeding truck, an angry supervisor, or a lump in the breast. Fear is focused on the threatening object, person, or situation. When that has been removed or dealt with, the fear subsides. Anxiety is a more generalized feeling, not so well focused. Anxiety may show itself in a vague sense of dread, a feeling of general apprehension, or a tendency to be fearful in any situation. Since all of us have both fears and anxiety, an illness as serious as heart disease can arouse both the objective response to danger as well as a more pervasive underlying dread.

No doubt the underlying fear in all life-threatening illness is the fear of death itself. "Will I survive this episode? How much longer can I expect to live?" But a number of other fears of lesser magnitude accompany the fear of death. *How* will I survive? What kind of life lies ahead of me? Will I be able to go back to work? Will I really be capable of doing my job satisfactorily? Do I have enough insurance to cover the costs of my hospitalization? Do I have enough sick time to take care of my convalescence? Is the doctor going to tell me that I have to have an operation? Will I be able to support my family when this is all over? Will I be able to play golf once again? Will I be able to enjoy sex? Will people think of me as an invalid? These questions represent only a few of the many fears with which the heart patient may have to deal.

Figure 1
The Spiritual Crisis of Serious Illness

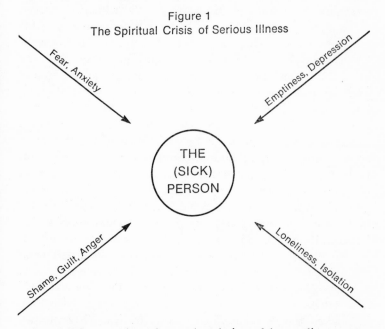

In addition to these fears, the victim of heart disease may also experience a kind of general apprehension or dread that is not so clearly focused on the illness itself, but colors his entire attitude towards himself, other people, and the world at large. Sometimes this anxiety has its roots in early child-hood experiences. Since to be seriously ill usually places us in a state of dependence, vulnerability, and helplessness similar to that of childhood, it is not surprising that many unrealistic fears and fantasies of childhood may be reawakened within us. All we need to do to understand this is to remember the first time we slept in a room by ourselves, or our first experience getting lost from our parents.

An unusual example of this is the case of a man in his middle thirties who was admitted to the hospital for evaluation of a heart condition. After thorough studies, the medical team was ready to send him home, having concluded that his disease could be successfully managed by medication and some reasonable limitation of his activity. The patient, however, was so anxious he could not sleep for more than ten to fifteen minutes at a time. Whenever he lay down to sleep, he felt as though everything was "turning grey" and "closing in" on him, and he became so afraid he had to get up and pace up and down the hall. His agitation was making it impossible for him to get the rest which his heart demanded.

Since the patient had expressed some religious concern, a chaplain was called to see if he could help relieve the man's extreme anxiety. In his initial conversation with the patient he learned that several family members had died recently of heart disease. Clearly there was some reason for this person to be afraid, and to wonder, "Am I going to be next?" Yet the physicians had done everything possible to reassure him that his condition was not an immediate threat to his life. It seemed that there had to be more behind his recurrent panic than simple fear. Playing a hunch, the chaplain asked, "Did you ever lose anyone close to you when you were a child?" The patient nodded, and his eyes filled with tears. "Who was it?" asked the chaplain. The patient replied, "My mother. She died in a mental hospital when I was seven years old." "That must have been very painful for you," the chaplain responded.

The patient went on to tell a strange and frightening

story. His mother had been emotionally disturbed for quite some time before she was finally committed to a hospital. One afternoon while the father was at work, the mother had put the children down for their afternoon naps. She had locked the doors, sealed the windows, turned on the gas, and then lay down to die with her children. Fortunately someone had come and gained entrance to the house before she and the children were completely overcome. The chaplain was struck by the resemblance between this experience and the patient's earlier description of things turning grey and closing in on him whenever he lay down to sleep. "You must have been terribly frightened," he observed. "No," said the patient, "I don't remember feeling frightened at all." But when he had finished the story, the patient remarked, "I don't tell this to very many people." Then his mood seemed visibly to lift, and he became more relaxed. "You know, I feel better now." Two days later he was able to go home. In addition to the normal and realistic fears arising from his disease, his profound anxiety resulting from this terrifying experience of his childhood, was causing him to be much more afraid of his disease than he needed to be. This anxiety had to be relived by his retelling the painful story before he could begin to deal constructively with his condition.

The spiritual integrity of the seriously ill person is threatened not only by fear and anxiety, but also by feelings of *shame* and *guilt*. A group of church members were discussing what they expected of a pastor. Most of them assigned a very high priority to hospital calling. One member of the group, a farmer in his early thirties, remarked that if he were in the hospital, the last thing he would want his pastor to do would be to visit him. When asked why he felt this way he replied, "I would feel embarrassed about having to be in the hospital, and I wouldn't want to see any of my friends and neighbors while I was there." Clearly he had somehow acquired the attitude that it was shameful to be sick! This feeling may be more common than we realize. Being sick means being idle, being weak, and having to be waited on by others. Since for most of us a large part of our self-esteem rests on being active, strong, and self-reliant, it is not strange that a serious illness should arouse some feelings of embarrassment and shame. The young farmer didn't want his friends or his pastor to see him in what he imagined to be a humiliating position.

Guilt is also a very common enemy to the person overtaken by serious illness. "Why did this happen to me?" and "What did I do to deserve this?" are questions that will be heard again and again by anyone who works with persons in the hospital. Sometimes the feeling conveyed is not so much that of guilt as of anger and protest. What the sick person is saying is, "It isn't fair that this has happened to me! I haven't done anything to deserve this!" Studies of dying patients have made us aware of the fact that anger is a very common response to the knowledge that one is going to die. It is a natural accompaniment of the "fight" response by which the human organism seeks to defend itself from attack. My own experience as a hospital chaplain suggests that anger is a common emotional response not just to terminal illness, but to *any* serious health problem. Further, it seems for some persons to be an alternative to guilt: those who are angry about their illness are less apt to feel guilty, and vice versa.

But what about guilt? Why is it that so many people do interpret their illness as punishment? There are of course numerous biblical passages which suggest that sickness is a consequence of sin:

> There is no soundness in my flesh
>   because of thy indignation;
> there is no health in my bones
>   because of my sin.
>   PSALM 38:3

> Some were sick through their sinful ways,
>   and because of their iniquities
>   suffered affliction.
>   PSALM 107:17

But there are many other passages which clearly deny that *all* sickness can be construed as punishment.

> As he passed by, he saw a man blind from his birth. And his disciples asked him, "Rabbi, who sinned, this man or his parents, that he was born blind?" Jesus answered, "It was not that this man sinned, or his parents, but that the works of God might be made manifest in him."
>
> JOHN 9:1-3

Why do so many people nevertheless feel guilty when they become seriously ill?

Some people are aware of ways in which they have contributed to their own illness. Those suffering from certain forms of heart disease may have good reason for holding themselves partly responsible for their condition. Excessive smoking, a diet over-rich in fats or sugars, lack of regular daily exercise, untreated hypertension, a harried, hurried, and highly competitive life-style all combine to increase the risk of coronary heart disease. In other words, the guilt that some people feel over their illness may be a realistic and legitimate assessment of their own history of irresponsibility to their bodies. When this is the case it will do little good for a kind friend, relative, or pastor to brush it aside with a reassuring comment. It will need to be faced honestly by the sick person with the help of a trusted confidant.

Another source of guilt should also be noted. Richard Gardner, a psychiatrist, has pointed out that the only alternative some people may be able to see to the view that illness is punishment is the view that it happens accidentally and is therefore completely unpredictable. Sickness viewed as punishment assumes that life is under the governance of a just and wise God who distributes happiness and misery in exact correspondence to each person's deserts. To take the view that sickness is purely accidental may suggest to such people that they live in an ungoverned universe where events are random, chaotic, and finally meaningless. For such persons, the latter alternative may be much more frightening than the former. Further, if one is sick because of some sin, one can perhaps overcome the sickness by recognizing the nature of the offense and correcting his subsequent behavior. If no such connection is seen between sin and sickness, the person may feel helpless to alter his circumstances or influence the outcome of his disease in any way.

A third threat to the spiritual well-being of the sick person comes from feelings of *emptiness* and *depression* which result from the loss of hope and meaningful purpose in life. Often we identify ourselves by our activity. If asked, "Who are you?" we reply by describing what we do for a living. "I'm a teacher . . . I'm a farmer . . . I drive a truck . . . I'm a housewife." The person who becomes seriously ill with heart disease is cut off from his or her normal activity, at least for the time being, and forced into a comparatively passive mode of existence. Life no longer consists of doing, but of having things done to or for oneself. One does not so much act as allow oneself to be *acted upon*. Hurrying and caring for others gives way to waiting and being cared for. All of this can have disastrous effects on the mental state of the sick person. Boredom sets in; it is hard to keep track of the days of the week because each is monotonously like the other. One feels useless, unproductive, and wonders, "Will I ever be any good for anything again?"

It is my impression that as a group, heart patients are even more vulnerable than other sick people to these feelings, because they are even more committed than the average person to a life of "doing." Hence they are all the more likely to fret at being deprived of their normal activities, and at having to adopt a passive, waiting response to their illness. Boredom and restlessness may stalk them through the weeks of convalescence after a serious episode; their greatest desire is to get back to work and to feel productive and useful once more. Their chief frustration is the slowness of their progress toward this goal.

The fourth arrow in our diagram represents the forces of

loneliness, isolation, and *depersonalization.* Any illness tends to isolate people from their community and family. The more serious the illness, the greater the degree of isolation that accompanies it. If we have a bad cold, we may stay home from work for several days; this is a very mild and temporary degree of isolation. If we have pneumonia, we may have to go to a hospital. Now we are isolated not only from those with whom we work, but to some extent from our family as well. The person who suffers a heart attack may be placed in an intensive or coronary care unit, where even family members are allowed to visit only briefly and at designated intervals. The greater the degree of illness, the more it shuts the person off from the normal stream of activities and pattern of relationships.

There are of course other factors that make serious illness a lonely experience. Pain and discomfort are very individual and subjective factors. No one can feel them for us or with us. In a real sense, the person in pain is alone in his or her pain, walled off from others by an experience that can be described but not directly shared. Moreover, many people hesitate to speak of their discomfort because they feel the need to appear brave, or because they do not wish to acquire the reputation of a complainer. The seriously ill person is so dependent on others that often he is reluctant to do or say anything that might offend those who provide care. Hospital procedure also contributes to the sense of isolation through its tendency to depersonalize the sufferer. In many hospitals, when the patient is admitted the first thing that is done is to assign him a hospital number (his name is no longer a significant mark of his personal identity) and to issue him a hospital gown that looks exactly like that worn by every other patient in the hospital. Before long his body will be subjected to numerous tests, procedures and examinations in which it will be prodded, thumped, probed, and scrutinized with clinical detachment by various members of the health care team. His privacy will be invaded by countless questions concerning the intimate details of his personal life. Occasionally members of the medical team may even discuss him in the third person as though he were not present. Much of this —though not all—is no doubt necessary, an unavoidable consequence of modern medical technology. One would hardly want physicians to become so personally involved in one's care that they are no longer capable of reaching a diagnosis with some degree of scientific detachment. Nevertheless, the result may be an assault on the sense of identity and self-worth of the sick person, who can be made to feel as though he were a nobody, a non-person.

Religious Responses to Illness

Having examined some of the ways in which serious illness may produce a spiritual crisis, we must now ask, "How may religious faith lead a person to deal with this crisis?" At least four different kinds of religious response are possible to the spiritual crisis of illness.

First, religious faith may lead some people to *deny* the reality of the threat which they face, or to *minimize* the seriousness of that threat. Some persons feel that their faith should make them immune to fear, guilt, depression or loneliness, that as believers they should be far beyond such normal human feelings. This attitude leads a few people to reject medical care entirely, and to seek healing through religious or spiritual means such as prayer, the laying on of hands, or what the followers of Mary Baker Eddy call "divine Science." Indeed Christian Science teaches that the physical affirmation of disease must always be countered by mental denial. Such a radical response to sickness is unusual. What is more common is to find the person playing down the painful or distressing aspects of his or her illness. An elderly widow who had been hospitalized numerous times for congestive heart failure was visited by a hospital chaplain. A devout adherent of a small and strict Protestant denomination, and hospitalized 100 miles from her home, she appeared to the chaplain to be an intensely lonely person. Frequently during their conversations she would sigh in a dejected way and say, "All I have left now is my Lord." But whenever the chaplain tried to reflect her mood by responding, "You must be very lonely at times," she would invariably deny it. "Oh no, I'm never lonely. My Lord is always with me." She was not only unable to acknowledge her very human longing for companionship and affection, she was also unwilling to cooperate with the physicians who were treating her illness. Although she had been warned repeatedly of the consequences, she refused to follow the low-salt and fluid-restricted diet on which her life depended. She was using her rather rigid style of believing in a powerful attempt to insulate herself from the pain of her loneliness. As a result she resisted both medical and spiritual help when they were offered.

A second way in which religious faith may function in the crisis of illness is to *intensify* the painful and threatening aspects of the situation. Fear and anxiety may be augmented by images of a wrathful deity and of judgment to come. Guilt may be upheld by belief in a God who rewards good behavior with health and uses disease to punish the disobedient. Depression may be observed among persons whose religious life is almost exclusively activist and service-oriented, and upon whom illness imposes a passive, dependent role. Separation from one's fellow-believers can intensify the sense of isolation as it did for the elderly widow described above.

Third, religious faith may be employed to *reduce* the intensity of fear, loneliness, or guilt and to *relieve* their painful sting. A patient facing open heart surgery urgently requested the Sacrament of Baptism prior to his operation. In seeking to assess the level of understanding of the person, the minister asked why it was so important to him to receive Baptism at this time. The reply came in words similar to the following: "The doctor has told me that this is a *very* serious operation, and . . . well . . . you just never know what may happen." When the sacrament had been administered, the patient seemed almost visibly relieved of tension. In this situation a religious rite was employed to reduce the intense anxiety that was felt by a person confronting the possibility of death. More than a few of the requests which a hospital chaplain receives involve a similar use of religious beliefs and symbols: to provide relief from a burden of anxiety, guilt, or depression which would otherwise be intolerable.

The fourth type of religious response to the crisis of illness is shown in Figure 2. Just as the sick person is attacked from without by powerful threats to his emotional and spiritual well-being, so it is possible at times for resources to be mobilized which buttress the person from within, and enable him to withstand the outward pressures of a life situation threatened by illness. The person is able to face and to bear anxiety, guilt, despair, and isolation without denying, minimizing or reducing their impact, by virtue of powers which enable him to continue to affirm his own being, his confidence in other persons, and the meaningfulness of his existence with courage and dignity.

Releasing Spiritual Resources

In response to anxiety and fear, the person may rediscover and gain access to deeper *faith*. The word is used with many shades of meaning. To one person, the word faith means, "I believe in God," while to another it means, "I'm sure I'm going to get well." Often patients in the hospital declare that they have faith in their doctor, meaning that they are confident of his skill and dedication. For some people the term "faith" carries magical overtones; they seek the proper formula or ritual that will "put God to work" for them and bring healing within their grasp. For others, faith involves some kind of bargain with the Divine: "O Lord, if you will help me get well, I promise that I will leave a share of my estate to medical research." But the faith which provides inner strength to bear and withstand the anxiety of illness goes beyond these levels. It is more like what the psychologist Erik Erikson calls "basic trust," an unyielding confidence that no matter what may come, one will be given the courage to see it through; that in spite of pain, loss, and even death itself, one's being will be graciously fulfilled by the Giver of Life. In the Hebrew Scriptures this faith finds expression in the declaration of the psalmist:

> God is our refuge and strength,
>> a very present help in trouble.
> Therefore we will not fear though the earth
>> should change,
>> though the mountains shake in the heart
>> of the sea.

PSALM 46:1-2

Likewise in the New Testament the apostle Paul sets forth his confidence

> that neither death nor life, nor angels, nor principalities, nor things present, nor things to come, nor powers, nor height, nor depth, nor anything else in all creation, will be able to separate us from the love of God in Christ Jesus our Lord.

ROMANS 8:38-39

Such faith is grounded in a relationship of trust in a Reality which is greater and more enduring than one's own fragile self, which cares for and seeks to complete the broken and fragmentary existence of each individual person. Not infrequently one hears this faith expressed by a patient facing a necessary but risky hospital procedure in words such as these:

> Oh yes, I have to admit I'm kind of nervous. I guess anybody would be. But I'm not really afraid. I have confidence in my doctors. Most of all, I know that God is with me. And I'm sure that whatever happens, it will be all right.

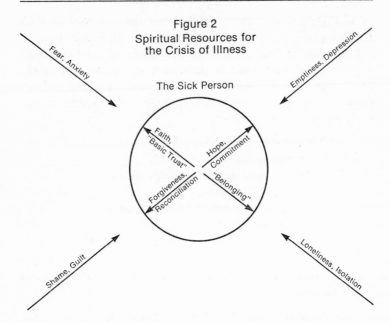

Figure 2
Spiritual Resources for
the Crisis of Illness

For persons who feel some significant degree of guilt, shame, or anger in connection with their illness, some *forgiveness* or *reconciliation* is appropriate. If the guilt is experienced primarily in relation to God, a rite of confession and absolution may provide a means for its resolution. Unlike Catholics, Protestants have no sacrament of confession. For many, however, the Sacrament of the Lord's Supper may bear this meaning, especially if the way is prepared beforehand by thoughtful pastoral conversation. Other persons will find release from guilt not through any formal rite, but by honestly opening their lives to another person whom they trust, whether it be a pastor or priest; a nurse, social worker or physician; or a friend, relative or fellow-patient. Where the sense of guilt involves strained or broken relationships, a frank exploration of the issues that have caused the break may need to be held with those from whom the person has become estranged.

Sometimes the predominant feeling is not guilt but anger. When this is the case it is important to identify the sources or the object of the anger. Many people are very uncomfortable dealing with anger and are reluctant to express it openly and directly. This is especially true of the seriously ill person, who does not want to risk offending any of those on whom he or she depends for essential care. Anger may arise at hospital procedures or policies: a long wait for an examination which results in the patient's missing lunch, or a delay in receiving a crucial laboratory report are examples. In such cases, frank complaints can sometimes initiate changes in hospital practices which will enhance the comfort and convenience of the patient. Sometimes the anger may be toward a particular member of the staff who seems inconsiderate of the patient's feelings or needs. It is usually helpful to bring this to the attention of the person involved, to allow any misunderstandings to be cleared up and to enable the staff member to evaluate and correct his or her behavior if it has been inappropriate. Sometimes the patient's anger arises from the disease itself. When this is the case, it is important that the patient, family members and staff recognize it. Not only does the pinpointing of the source help to prevent the anger from spilling over into generalized irritability and crabbiness, but the anger may become a valuable adjunct in therapy if it can be channeled toward resisting or overcoming the disease. Some persons are angry not so much at others or their disease, but at a God who appears to have abandoned them to weakness and pain. Such persons can be reminded that genuine faith is not incompatible with the spirit of complaint and protest, as numerous psalms attest.

> How long, O Lord? Wilt thou forget me for ever?
> How long wilt thou hide thy face from me?
> How long must I bear pain in my soul,
> And have sorrow in my heart all the day?
>
> PSALM 13:1-2

Prayers of protest may be addressed with boldness to a God who does not retaliate against those who are angry at him, but takes the complaints of his servants seriously and embraces them within his all-inclusive love.

Where shame is a predominant feeling, it may be necessary for the sick person to become reconciled to, even to forgive, the body which has let him or her down by becoming ill. For many of us, one of the most difficult challenges which illness presents is to learn to accept ourselves as weak, needy, vulnerable, and dependent beings. We value ourselves as persons of worth only so long as we are able to fulfill our expectations of being strong, healthy, active, and self-reliant; moreover we assume that others value us in the same way we value ourselves. What we have to learn is that our worth does not depend on our degree of health, and that even when we are weak and needy we are nevertheless persons of sacred worth. The apostle Paul seems to have experienced such a reconciliation to his own infirmity.

> And to keep me from being too elated by the abundance of revelations, a thorn was given me in the flesh, a messenger of Satan, to harass me, to keep me from being too elated. Three times I besought the Lord about this, that it should leave me, but he said to me, "My grace is sufficient for you, for my power is made perfect in weakness." . . . For the sake of Christ, then, I am content with weaknesses, insults, hardships, persecutions, and calamities; for when I am weak, then I am strong.
>
> 2 CORINTHIANS 12:7-9a, 10

For those who are assaulted by a sense of emptiness, meaninglessness and depression as a result of illness, *hope* is an essential inner resource. Both Elisabeth Kübler-Ross in her study of dying patients, and Viktor Frankl in his account of life in a Nazi concentration camp have stressed the vital role of hope. But hope, like faith, exists in many different dimensions. The simplest of these for the sick person is the hope of recovery from illness. But what if full recovery is uncertain, or even impossible? The person whose functional heart capacity is permanently impaired may need encouragement and assistance in rethinking his or her life-goals, and in reordering his or her priorities, so that a realistic hope may be maintained. Frankl describes the interplay of three different modes of value which underlie hope in the life of the person. Most of us spend a substantial portion of our lives in the pursuit of *creative* values, making and doing, producing and accumulating. Planting a garden, teaching a class, repairing a car, painting a house, writing a book, winning the award as salesman-of-the-year — all are examples of creative values. Although many of our hopes are directed toward the realization of creative values, not all of life can be lived in the active mode: some of it must necessarily be passive.

In addition to creative values, there must also be *experiential* values, those which revolve around receiving, appreciating, and enjoying. Watching a sunset, listening to a symphony, sharing in meaningful conversation with a friend are examples of experiential values. Still a third category of values, called *existential,* includes the meaning that may be found in suffering when suffering is unavoidable. The person whose illness is life-altering in the sense that it brings with it the diminution of strength and necessitates more limited physical activity or social responsibility will need to invest less of his life in creative values, and more in experiential and existential. An excellent example of this process can be found in *The Year of My Rebirth,* by the Kentucky poet and novelist Jesse Stuart. The book is a diary which the author kept during his own recovery from a near-fatal heart attack, and chronicles his own rediscovery of a slower pace for his life and a more relaxed, receptive, and appreciative attitude toward nature and other people.

When depression occurs, it seldom seems helpful to try to talk the person out of it. What begins as a well-meaning attempt to cheer the person up may quickly descend into an argument: "Just think how much you have to be thankful for. You're alive, you have a good home, a loving family. Lots of people are worse off than you!" Almost invariably, the result of this kind of a conversation (or monolog) is not that the sick person feels less depressed, but that he or she feels even more depressed, because it is clear now that no one can really understand how bad things seem! Superficial reassurance is likewise seldom helpful: "Don't worry—one of these days you'll be out of the hospital and as good as new." The real and often painful changes and losses that illness brings must be faced without evasion, whether these involve changes in diet and exercise habits, decreased responsibilities at work, early retirement due to disability, or even a greatly reduced life-expectancy.

Perhaps the most significant way in which religious faith can arouse hope is by enlisting the commitment of the person to something or someone beyond the narrow boundaries of the self. When life is understood as a vocation involving service to a cause, an ideal, a community, or above all to God himself, then hope is sustained by a continuing sense of purpose in one's existence. For the genuinely religious person, the meaningfulness of life is not only a gift but also a task to be taken up daily and fulfilled. As Frankl reports, those prisoners in the concentration camps who came to believe that they had nothing more to expect from life had to learn that what really mattered was not what *they* expected from life, but what *life* expected of them! Their way of asking the question had to be changed from, "What meaning does life hold for me now?" to "What meaning will I *give* to my life now?" Likewise the victim of heart disease who struggles with a sense of emptiness and hopelessness may be enabled through vital religious faith to see his life as a continuing task that requires completion for the sake of others, and above all for the sake of God.

The last of the inner buttressing forces on our diagram is

the sense of *belonging,* which can overcome the threat of isolation and depersonalization. The sense of belonging may be nourished in a number of ways. Most seriously ill persons value greatly any cards, letters, messages, or phone calls from friends and family. Visitors are also appreciated, especially when they keep their visits brief and show consideration for the physical and emotional tolerance of the patient. Persons in the hospital frequently find comfort also in the presence of fellow-sufferers. It is not unusual to hear words such as the following: "You just can't feel sorry for yourself here. All you have to do is look around you to see there are lots of people who have it just as hard as you." What is supportive is the knowledge that one is not alone in sickness, but shares in a wider community of suffering.

In fact, the most significant and immediately helpful spiritual resource to those who are afflicted with serious illness consists of *other people*—people who care and who are able to express their caring sensitively and effectively. Any person may do this, professional or non-professional, providing he or she can relate to the sick person with honesty, understanding, and acceptance. A sense of belonging is nurtured in relationships in which the helping person seeks actively to listen; to listen not only for ideas and information but for subtle nuances of feeling, to listen not only for the words, but also for the "music" of the message. The sensitive listener tries not so much to change the attitude or outlook of the speaker, as to understand why and how the speaker sees things in his or her particular way. Yet, understanding is frequently the one thing that will make possible a change of attitude, for it breaks through the isolating walls of silence that so often surround the sufferer.

Religious faith can offer powerful support and confirmation for a sense of belonging. The religious person is conscious of belonging not just to family, friends and community, but to a fellowship of faith which extends far beyond his or her immediate network of relationships both in time and space.

> So then you are no longer strangers and sojourners, but you are fellow citizens with the saints and members of the household of God.
>
> EPHESIANS 2:19

In this connection it is often immeasurably strengthening to the sick person to know that others are praying for him or her, for these prayers are an expression not only of their personal caring but also of the sufferer's membership in "the communion of saints." Moreover, the religious person knows that he or she belongs to the God whom this community worships, and whose love is the foundation of its existence. No circumstances can ever completely separate us from this God.

> Whither shall I go from thy Spirit?
>   Or whither shall I flee from thy presence?
> If I ascend to heaven, thou are there!
>   If I make my bed in Sheol, thou art there!
> If I take the wings of the morning
>   and dwell in the uttermost parts of the sea,
> even there thy hand shall lead me,
>   and thy right hand shall hold me.
>
> PSALM 139:7-10

Such a conviction brings access to powerful inner resources which can enable the heart patient to resist the corrosive forces of isolation and depersonalization.

One final word of caution, however. The person whose faith supplies this kind of inner buttressing is not the person who embraces religion primarily for the benefits it is thought to offer. The person whose faith in time of serious illness provides strength to resist and overcome anxiety, guilt, depression, and loneliness does not believe primarily in order to gain access to the peace and strength which faith supplies, but rather because he is convinced that the object of his faith is in some deep and lasting sense true and trustworthy. He worships God not simply as the source from whom all earthly blessings flow, but as the one supreme reality alone worthy of adoration and commitment. There is about such faith a self-forgetful, self-transcending quality which is reflected in the familiar prayer of St. Francis of Assisi:

> *Lord, make me an instrument of your peace. Where there is hatred let me sow love; where there is injury, pardon; where there is discord, union; where there is doubt, faith; where there is despair, hope; where there is darkness, light; and where there is sadness, joy.*

> *O Divine Master, grant that I may not so much seek to be consoled, as to console; to be understood as to understand; to be loved, as to love. For it is in giving that we receive, it is in pardoning that we are pardoned, and it is in dying that we are born to eternal life. Amen.*

Notes

1. Thomas P. Hackett and Ned H. Cassem, "Psychological Reactions to Life-Threatening Illness: Acute Myocardial Infarction," in *Psychological Aspects of Stress*, ed. by Harry S. Abram, Springfield, Illinois, Charles C. Thomas, 1970, pp. 29-43.

2. *The Year of My Rebirth*, New York, McGraw Hill, 1956, pp. 10-11.

3. E. L. Cay, N. Vetter, A. E. Philip and P. Dugard, "Psychological Status During Recovery from an Acute Heart Attack," *Journal of Psychosomatic Research*, 16:5 (1972) pp. 425-435.

4. M. Skelton and J. Dominian, "Psychological Stress in Wives of Patients with Myocardial Infarction," *British Medical Journal*, 14 April, 1973, pp. 101-103.

5. Jess Lair and Jacqueline Carey Lair, *"Hey God, What Do I Do Now?"* Garden City, New York, Doubleday, 1973, pp. 17 ff.

119

6. Richard R. Miles, "Sexual Intercourse and the Cardiac Patient," in *Stress and the Heart*, ed. by Robert S. Eliot, Mount Kisco, New York, Futura, 1974, pp. 197-204.

7. Lenore R. Zohman and Jerome Tobis, *Cardiac Rehabilitation*, New York, Grune and Stratton, 1970, p. 144.

8. *Ibid.*, pp. 115-131.

9. *"I Ain't Much, Baby, But I'm All I've Got,"* Garden City, New York, Doubleday, 1969, p. 12.

10. *Op. cit.*

11. Elizabeth Kelleher, *A Descriptive Study of the Feeling State of Disturbance in Patients Awaiting Heart Surgery*, M.A. Thesis, Iowa City, Iowa: State University of Iowa, 1968.

12. Kenneth A. Frank, Stanley S. Heller, and Donald S. Kornfeld, "A Survey of Adjustment to Cardiac Surgery," *Archives of Internal Medicine*, V. 130 (November, 1972), pp. 735-738.

13. Carolyn Ruth Richardson, *An Exploratory Study to Identify Problems Perceived by the Cardiac Surgery Patient During Early Convalescence at Home*, M.A. Thesis, Iowa City, Iowa: University of Iowa, 1975, pp. 143, 161-163.

14. Madeline Petrillo and Sirgay Sanger, *Emotional Care of Hospitalized Children*, Philadelphia, J. B. Lippincott Company, 1972, pp. 178-185. On this topic see also Emma Plank, *Working with Children in Hospitals*, Cleveland, The Press of Case Western Reserve University, 1962.

For Further Reading

The American Heart Association Cookbook, edited by Ruthe Eshleman and Mary Winston. New and expanded edition. New York, David McKay, 1975.

A varied and imaginative collection of recipes and suggestions for low-fat, low-cholesterol meals, this book can help transform weight control into a culinary adventure.

Friedman, Meyer, and Ray H. Rosenman, *Type A Behavior and Your Heart,* Greenwich, Connecticut, Fawcett, 1974.

This very readable book by two of the nation's leading cardiologists is available in an inexpensive paperback edition. It presents evidence which the authors' research has accumulated linking coronary heart disease to a particular pattern of behavior and personality, and offers specific guidelines for the prevention of heart disease, including dietary advice.

121

Heart Attack! What Now? Atlanta, Georgia Heart Association, 1972.

> The nature, causes, symptoms and consequences of heart attacks are explained in clear and simple terms in this booklet, which some hospitals give to all coronary patients at the time they are discharged. Practical guidelines are offered concerning diet, exercise, activity, and rest for the person recovering from a heart attack. One section includes spaces where the physician may write specific instructions for the individual patient.

Kelly, Orville, with Randall Becker, *Make Today Count,* New York, Delacourte, 1975.

> The story of how the author, a cancer patient, learned to live with his own life-threatening illness, and is helping other persons faced with a similar task.

Kesten, Yehuda, *Diary of a Heart Patient,* New York, McGraw-Hill, 1968.

> An Israeli journalist suffering from Marfan's syndrome recounts his experience in being operated on twice by Dr. Michael DeBakey of Houston.

Lair, Jess, and Jacqueline Carey Lair, *"Hey God, What Should I Do Now?",* Garden City, New York, Doubleday, 1973.

> An engrossing account of one man's heart attack, its impact on his family, and the new directions in his personal and professional life which emerged from the experience. Alternate chapters are written by husband and wife, thus showing two different perspectives on the same series of events. Available in paperback.

Lawton, George, *Straight to the Heart,* New York, International Universities Press, 1956.

Still another personal experience, this time by a psychotherapist who underwent surgery for repair of a defective aortic valve. Readers of this book should note that it was written during the very early days of open heart surgery, and bear in mind that the past two decades have seen dramatic advances in the surgical treatment of heart disease.

Lynch, James J. *The Broken Heart: The Medical Consequences of Loneliness.* New York, Basic Books, 1977.

Dr. Lynch, a leading specialist in psychosomatic medicine at the University of Maryland School of Medicine, shows that the incidence of premature death from heart disease is significantly higher among persons who lack love and companionship — the widowed, divorced and separated; the old and the single young living alone; and children from broken homes.

Petrillo, Madeline, and Sirgay Sanger, *Emotional Care of Hospitalized Children,* Philadelphia, Lippincott, 1972.

Written by a pediatric nurse and a child psychiatrist for the guidance of health care professionals, this book nevertheless contains much information of interest and value to parents whose child must undergo hospitalization and surgery.

Phibbs, Brendan, *The Human Heart,* with contributions by Lane D. Craddock, 3rd edition, St. Louis, Mosley, 1975.

A wealth of information concerning the structure and function of the heart and the types, symptoms, causes, diagnosis and treatment of heart disease is presented in clear and readable language in this book, which was written by a physician for the non-medical person.

Plank, Emma, *Working with Children in Hospitals,* Cleveland, The Press of Western Reserve University, 1962.

A slim volume intended for professional health care workers. Parents too might benefit from reading the excellent brief chapters on admitting children to the hospital, relationships between children within the hospital, and preparing for and working through feelings after surgery.

Ross, John Jr., and Robert A. O'Rourke, *Understanding the Heart and Its Diseases,* New York, McGraw, 1976.

This book was written to provide paramedical health professionals and lay persons with a working knowledge of heart disease. In addition to describing the effects of disease on the heart, the authors, both physicians, discuss diagnostic procedures, the role of medication and surgery in the treatment of heart problems, and the various risk factors which contribute to heart disease.

Scheingold, Lee Dreisinger, and Nathaniel Wagner, *Sound Sex and the Aging Heart,* New York, Human Sciences, 1974.

Based on recent research in both sexual behavior and heart disease, this book stresses the continuing possibility of meaningful sexual relationships for persons with cardiac problems. Though some readers may take exception to the "rational and non-moralistic" value perspective on sex which the authors assume, the information presented here is most valuable.

Stuart, Jesse, *The Year of My Rebirth,* New York, McGraw-Hill, 1956.

Written by a well-known novelist and poet, this book is a spiritual diary of the author's recovery from a near-fatal heart attack, and tells of his rediscovery of self, family, friends, nature, and God during his year of convalescence.